Nobody is better positioned to speak with both informed authority and compassion about the wrenching problem of establishing genuine health care for all Americans. His lively and seasoned presentation will appeal to every interested reader. More to the point, perhaps, is the fact that Morris's words should be required reading for every single person—politician, cleric, social worker, insurance executive, physician, or medical administrator—whose work in any way impacts health in this country.

PHYLLIS TICKLE, author of *The Great Emergence*

I have seen many faith-based programs around the world, and the Church Health Center is one of the most impressive. So impressive, in fact, that I made it the centerpiece of a chapter in a book called *What Good Is God?* Scott Morris answers that question not with abstract argument but with creative, compassionate service. His story is thrilling, and if more people followed his example the contentious health care debate would fall silent.

PHILIP YANCEY, author of
What's So Amazing about Grace and *The Jesus I Never Knew*

Dr. Morris has done the seemingly impossible—created a thriving health care clinic for the working uninsured, funded by volunteers and the faith community. His vision, as well as his passion for redefining wellness, completely changes the paradigm of how we look at health care. This book is a must read for everyone of faith.

HAROLD G. KOENIG, M.D., Director of Center for Spirituality,
Theology, and Health, Duke University Medical Center

This clear, accessible book invites us to "clothe" ourselves and our medical practice in the generous truth of the gospel. This book is a must because our old ways have failed and new ways rooted in holy truth are on offer.

WALTER BRUEGGEMANN, Professor Emeritus, Columbia Theological Seminary

Dr. Morris fully embodies the biblical mandate to "preach, teach, and heal," but words in this book are more healing than teaching or preaching. Buy several copies of this book, for there is much wisdom in these chapters that you will want to share with others.

REV. DR. DEBORAH L. PATTERSON, Executive Director of
International Parish Nurse Resource Center and Deaconess Parish Nurse Ministries

Health Care You Can Live With is good medicine for your mind, your body, and your soul. Apply its principles daily and you will transform your health.

DAVID STEVENS, M.D., M.A.
CEO, Christian Medical & Dental Associations

You won't find another book like this. While there are books on the politics of health care and books about spiritual life, there are few books that bring body and spirit together in such a down-to-earth way. Dr. Morris writes from years of experience providing health care for thousands of working people without health insurance. His stories alone are worth reading—but even more, you will find tangible ways to become healthier and more fully alive. He's not embarrassed to talk about faith nor is he naïve when he says that health is more than the absence of disease. It's not false advertising to say that this book can change your life.

REV. DR. BARBARA K. LUNDBLAD
Joe R. Engle Professor of Preaching,
Union Theological Seminary in New York City

Dr. Morris has a clear passion for people and a deep compassion for their wellness. He reminds us that God cares about the health care crisis, and He has already written the greatest plan for reformation on the planet.

CHANTEL HOBBS, author of *Never Say Diet, The One Day Way,*
and *Love Food & Live Well*

Reading this book is like sitting down for a consultation with a skilled doctor who is also just plain wise about life. Dr. Morris offers sage counsel on every page. Anyone who opens up this book will be informed, inspired and encouraged.

MARTIN B. COPENHAVER
Senior Pastor, Wellesley Congregational Church, Wellesley, Massachusetts
Coauthor, *This Odd and Wondrous Calling:*
The Public and Private Lives of Two Ministers

In *Health Care You Can Live With*, Dr. Morris guides us back to where "real health" begins and where we should have been heading all along—straight to God's Word. It's impossible to find abundant personal health or realize true national reform without the foundation of biblical principles. Not a new discovery, but the only way to recovery. Thankfully, Dr. Morris knows how to get there.

JIMMY PEÑA
New York Times bestselling author and founder of PrayFit.com

In *Healthcare You Can Live With*, Dr. Scott Morris reminds us of our responsibility to take care of those in our community as well as ourselves. He poignantly reminds us that good health is not just the absence of disease, but a way of life and an outreach to others. It is a refreshing and inspiring book that all community development leaders should read. Morris's principles serve as marching orders for a new community health movement.

LARRY JAMES
President and CEO, CitySquare (formerly Central Dallas Ministries)

Health Care
YOU CAN
LIVE
With

Discover Wholeness
in Body *and* Spirit

Dr. Scott Morris
with Susan Martins Miller

BARBOUR
PUBLISHING

© 2011 by G. Scott Morris

ISBN 978-1-61626-247-1

Cover photography: Murray Riss Photography

Published by Barbour Publishing, Inc., P.O. Box 719, Uhrichsville, Ohio 44683, www.barbourbooks.com

Our mission is to publish and distribute inspirational products offering exceptional value and biblical encouragement to the masses.

ecpa Member of the
Evangelical Christian
Publishers Association

Printed in the United States of America.

To those who bring joy to my life
and thereby improve my health,
especially Mary.

Acknowledgments

This book has been more than twenty years in its creation. It reflects my growing and evolving understanding of health during the life of the Church Health Center in Memphis, Tennessee. Literally hundreds of people have contributed ideas to the process. Some who are no longer alive or working with us had important insights. To all who have been a part of the creation of this work, I am grateful.

I am especially thankful for the directors of the Church Health Center and our Wellness staff, and for our volunteers and donors who make the work possible. Mike Sturdivant and Jenny Bartlett-Prescott have championed our process of integrated health, with key leadership from Mary Cay Oyler and her staff. Clinically, David Jennings and Mary Nell Ford have seen endless patients over the years while I was out raising money or running my mouth. Our entire medical staff has eagerly embraced a new way of providing health care to our patients. Karen Wright works as my administrative assistant and has been critical to many of the details in this process. Administratively, Ann Langston has stood beside me for twenty-five years with her love of our mission.

All of us are influenced by the thinking of others. For me, William Sloane Coffin remains my mentor. Today Gary Gunderson and Gary Shorb help me to see what is possible in God's imagination.

I am thankful to Barbour Publishing for proposing the writing of this book. Without their encouragement I would still be thinking of doing it. I am forever grateful to Barbour for introducing me to my cowriter, Susan Martins Miller. She is a brilliant writer with keen insight into the meaning of health and is now a true friend.

And my wife, Mary, who has a sharp mind for what can bring love into our lives, makes me laugh and look forward to every day.

Contents

)

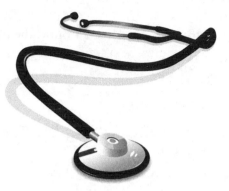

Introduction

The number one rule for a male doctor who examines a woman in a burqa is, "Stand back and don't touch."

This is more than a slight impediment to doctoring.

A Middle Eastern father brought his teenage daughter to see me. She wore the traditional clothing of her religiously conservative culture. After gathering as much information as I could through conversation, I knew I had to listen to her heart. I find this challenging from across the room. Thankfully the girl's father gave me permission to approach her with my stethoscope, and the girl started to adjust her burqa to allow me to use it. Removing the first layer revealed another thickness of black underneath. The folds parted again to expose a further swath of dark cloth. Finally she shifted most of the formless yardage out of the way, and I saw that next to her skin she wore a tee shirt like any American teenager.

KISS ME, I'M IRISH, it said.

Over the years, I've come to see the Church Health Center, where I practice family medicine, as the United Nations of Memphis. The working uninsured come to our open arms, whether U.S. citizens who move to Memphis for various reasons, lifelong

Tennessee natives, or immigrants from around the globe. They may find work in our city, but they don't have health insurance. The Church Health Center offers care, and where they come from is irrelevant. They come in need.

I first came to Memphis in 1986. I had no personal ties to Memphis and did not know anyone here. Having completed theological and medical education, I was determined to begin a health care ministry for the working poor. A lightbulb did not suddenly go on. I had dreamed of this for years as I slogged my way—sometimes impatiently—through the training that would make it possible. When the time came, I chose Memphis because historically it is one of the poorest major cities in the United States. I instigated relationships with St. John's United Methodist Church and Methodist University Hospital in Memphis, found an old house to rehab, and rolled up my sleeves. The next year, the doors of the Church Health Center opened with one doctor—me—and one nurse. We saw twelve patients the first day.

Today 55,000 people depend on us for their health care, and our Wellness facility welcomes 125,000 visitors a year. A staff of 220 people shares our ministry of healing and wellness. Hundreds more volunteer time and services. A network of medical specialists makes certain the uninsured working poor receive the same quality of health care as anyone with a Cadillac insurance plan. Fees slide on a scale based on income and family size.

So what sets us apart from other community clinics around the country?

The Church Health Center is fundamentally about the church. We care for our patients without relying on government funds because God calls the church to healing work. Jesus' life was about healing the whole person—body and spirit—and the church is Jesus in the world. Jesus' message is our message. Jesus' ministry is our ministry. Local congregations embrace this calling and help make our work possible. We have a budget of about $13 million a year, but the value of the health care we deliver is more than $100 million annually. And for every dollar we spend on treatment, our goal is to spend a dollar on prevention.

More than two decades of caring for the working uninsured have made one thing plain: Health care has to change. We have to do better than issue cards to give disadvantaged people access to a broken system. The church can choose to get involved by reclaiming the biblical mandate to bring healing. Individual congregations can choose to get involved by envisioning their role in the health of members and the community around them. Individual Christians can choose to get involved in changing health care by taking charge of their own health care. And it has nothing to do with what happens in Washington or who is president.

In the years that the Church Health Center has cared for people in Memphis, we've seen that two-thirds of our patients seek treatment for illness that healthier lifestyles can prevent or control. We realized that if we want to make a lasting difference in our patients' lives, the most effective strategy is encouraging overall wellness in body and spirit. We can put salve on what hurts at the moment, but what does that change? At a fundamental level, we must transform what the words *well* and *health* mean in the minds and hearts of most people. We've developed a "Model for Healthy Living" that communicates our heart for healing and wholeness in body and spirit.

Some of our patients teach us profound lessons, and we carry them into our own lives and relationships. As you read this book, you'll meet some of the people the Church Health Center serves. But this book is not just about the Church Health Center. It's about you. It's about your understanding of wellness. It's about your opportunity to experience lasting change in your own life.

And that is health care you can live with.

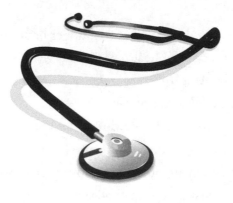

1

Health Care Is a Mess

*Nobody wants the government deciding
when you're going to die.*

W hen I was a fourth-year medical student, I met a witch doctor.

It wasn't easy. I spent a summer in Zimbabwe on a medical research project, and I took my curiosity about faith and healing with me on a few side trips. I wanted to meet a *nyanga*, a witch doctor, and I started asking about it as soon as my feet hit the ground in Zimbabwe. To meet a nyanga, you must have permission from a sort of nyanga association, so I asked permission. After two months of being turned down, I was running out of time. Finally I received permission just before I was due to return to the United States. I arranged to see a nyanga on a sugarcane plantation in southern Zimbabwe, right on the South Africa border. Dressed in overalls, he rode his bicycle in from his fields to meet with me in his house.

He took me into a back room and might as well have taken me into another world—candles, incense, a zebra skin, snakeskins.

I asked a few questions about the kinds of ailments people came to him with and how he treated them. In simple cases he pulled something from his shelves of herbs and roots, and in complicated cases he consulted his ancestral spirit. When this happened, the ancestor would take over the nyanga's body and tell him what kind of advice to give to the patient.

And then I asked my deepest question. In two months of working in Zimbabwe, I saw that people went to the nyanga and then immediately went to see a Western doctor. Clearly they believed Western medicine would help, but they always went to the nyanga first. Why?

The nyanga explained to me, "They come to me because I can tell them *why* they are sick."

Western doctors don't answer that question beyond a scientific-sounding answer about infections and disease. But that wasn't what the people in Zimbabwe were asking. They sought a spiritual answer to the question, "Why am I sick?" The nyanga generally would answer, "Because you failed to honor your ancestors," and tell patients what they should do to honor their ancestors. Then the people went to the doctor for medicine. They knew the Western doctor's medicine would make them physically well, but it would not stop the cause of the illness, which they did not believe was physical in origin.

The Zimbabweans who went to both the nyanga and the doctor knew you cannot separate body and spirit. Treating one without the other does not make you well. Don't get me wrong. I'm not saying every physical symptom results from some failure in a person's life. I *am* saying being well is about more than fixing a broken part of your body. The dominant approach to health care in the United States concerns broken bodies more than broken lives. We've developed systems that put people through hoops to get care but too often don't make them healthier.

Our system says, "Keep out."

Eve was forty-six when her life shattered. She had a good job, a happy family, and no significant history of illness. Then one night her chest started to hurt and she had a heart attack. An emergency bypass operation saved her life, but not the circulation in her legs. In a matter of days, surgeons amputated both her legs. During that one prolonged hospitalization, Eve used up her entire lifetime insurance benefit. Clearly she was going to have ongoing medical needs, so she applied for the state's version of Medicaid—and was turned down because she had health insurance. Somehow it didn't matter that she had no more benefits available under her policy.

Laura was two years old and asleep on her mother's lap when I met her. Laura had IGA deficiency, a disease of the immune system that made her susceptible to infections. Her mother, Jill, brought Laura in because she seemed to have a sinus infection. Jill calmly explained why she had come to the Church Health Center. A number of years earlier, her husband had had a relationship with a woman who later turned out to be infected with HIV. Now he was in the final stages of AIDS. When he became unable to work, Jill went back into the workforce. Getting a job—even without insurance benefits—meant she lost Medicaid coverage for herself and Laura, whose IGA deficiency required frequent medical attention.

Frank, a construction worker, fell off a ladder and hurt his shoulder. Even though he was in excruciating pain, he waited four days to see a doctor. It didn't take ten seconds to see what the problem was when he turned up in my exam room. An x-ray confirmed he had broken his collarbone and would need surgery to give him the use of his shoulder and arm. When I told him, he started to cry. "How can I afford to pay for this, especially when I can't work?"

Health care is a mess. People who need help can't always get it. Financial repercussions, not health repercussions, dominate their decisions. People like Eve and Laura and Frank are not so far away from you. Maybe you know somebody like this. Maybe you *are* somebody like this.

We have a health care system that says, "Keep out."

Keep out if you're poor, but not poor enough.

Keep out if you are not part of an employer's insurance plan.

Keep out if a computer can't automatically assign you neatly into a category.

Keep out if you are an illegal immigrant.

The question of health care reform pushes buttons in a lot of people—including me. If you're like most people, you wonder if all the talk about the health care crisis will bring any meaningful change. You have real-life questions and you want to know how legislation on such a major issue affects you and your family.

"Does this mean I can stop paying so much in premiums?"

"Are they trying to tell me what doctor I can see?"

"They're not going to reduce my coverage, are they?"

"Can I keep my kids on my policy?"

"How much is this going to cost me?"

"Why should I have to buy insurance if I don't want to?"

If we want lasting change in our health care system, however, we have to step back and ask the bigger questions.

Why is our health care system so broken in the first place? If we don't come face-to-face with what's broken, we can't fix it.

Who benefits from changes to the system? Will Eve and Laura and Frank be better off? Will you?

What does "health care" even mean?

Are more people going to be more well, or will more people simply have cards in their wallets?

Opinions on these questions are all over the board. You're going to find out what I think as you continue to read this book. History teaches many lessons, and it even sheds light on the kind of care doctors offer you. Whether you are employed or unemployed, insured or uninsured, disease free or living with a chronic condition, the "system" that comes out of our history affects *your* health care.

When the Church Health Center opened in 1987, twenty-six million Americans were uninsured. Today that number is close to fifty million, and the Congressional Budget Office estimates it could grow to fifty-four million by 2019. If all goes perfectly, the health care reform legislation signed into law in 2010 will be fully in place by 2019 and provide coverage for thirty-one million uninsured Americans. That still leaves twenty-three million people without insurance. On top of that, millions more—perhaps as many as a hundred million—will be underinsured as costs continue to rise. The government subsidies offered under the legislation are unlikely to be sufficient for full-blown insurance coverage. High deductibles essentially will mean the insurance plan has little effect on day-to-day health care. Steep out-of-pocket costs will still deter people from seeking care, even if they have insurance. If a plan does not reimburse physicians adequately, patients will have trouble finding doctors who accept the plan. And although a policy may kick in for a major illness, individuals still will bear costs they may never recover from financially. More than 60 percent of bankruptcies are related to medical bills, and three-fourths of these people have health insurance when they become ill.

People who cobble together income from multiple part-time jobs will remain uninsured. The new insurance plans in the 2010 legislation will remain out of reach financially. Certainly the immigrants among us will qualify for nothing. No matter what your views are on immigration, if someone who cleans our houses or cuts our lawns gets sick, we have an obligation to provide care.

We would all agree that the 2010 legislation launches us out into a brave new world of health care. Nothing about it is certain. Jesus said, "The poor will always be with you." So far he has been right. If he ever asks me, "Where were you when I was poor and sick?" I want to be able to answer, "I cared for you as best I could."

Doctors learn to keep out.

Doctors learn to practice medicine by taking a medical history and asking questions around the symptoms the patient describes. Ninety percent of the diagnosis is based on what the patient tells you. The doctor formulates an opinion about what is causing the problem and then performs a physical exam to collect more information about the suspected cause. Eventually diagnostic tests may confirm what the doctor thinks.

This process also says, "Keep out."

Keep out of my heart.

Keep out of my sorrow, my stress, my fatigue, my relationships.

Keep out of my private space. Just fix what hurts.

Eve, the woman who lost her legs after a heart attack, rocked continuously in her wheelchair the first time she came to see me in my practice at the Church Health Center. I tried to ignore it, but her husband asked, "Do you think you can do anything about her constant rocking?" I spoke to our pastoral counselor, and right away he said, "Often when people rock, it means they want to be held." He was absolutely right. Eve rocked herself because she felt deformed and unlovable and unable to interact physically with her family as she always had. When I talked to Eve's husband again, he immediately took her in his arms. She never rocked in my presence again.

Every day, every single day, doctors tell patients there's nothing wrong because they find no physical root for patient complaints. If we can't see a spot on a screen, a squiggle of dye on a test, a crack in an x-ray, or a level in the blood, then nothing is wrong. The person is "healthy." Whatever is amiss is not a matter for the health care system. Probably this happens to you. The doctor reassures you that you are "fine," but you wonder why you don't feel fine.

Plenty is wrong. Spiritual and emotional issues manifest in physical ways. But our health care system draws a line and says, "Keep out."

Palmer was ninety years old when he developed pneumonia and was admitted to the hospital in the middle of the night. When he stopped breathing, someone called a code, did CPR, resuscitated him, and put a tube down his throat to keep him breathing. For two weeks he lay in a bed in the intensive care unit, where they never turn the lights off, with a tube down his throat.

When a loved one finally asked, "Palmer, do you want a kiss?" this ninety-year-old man was ready to yank out the tube. The health care he needed at that moment—clearly he was dying—was not technology, but human contact. He wanted that kiss more than anything. But for two weeks the health care system had said, "Keep out," to his basic need.

Change means letting go.

Health care is a mess. People want change.

But to what?

Nobody wants the government deciding when you're going to die. That's not what health care reform is about. It's not about how many people carry a card imprinted with the name of an insurance company. It's not about living two weeks longer in a stark ICU. It's not about access to extreme technology in every small town.

Efforts at health care reform fail because they avoid the essential questions of wellness. The starting point is off kilter. Our health care system is built on the premise of waiting for people to break in some way and then come through our doors, where we will use our technological wizardry to fix them. "Access to health care" has come to mean having a card that lets you get through those doors. For too long we have accepted this definition of health care.

That's not health care. Caring for health means attending to the things that keep you well long before you break and need the door to technology. And believe it or not, doctors are only one part of true health care.

Change means getting used to the unfamiliar. For many people it's easier to clutch a tight fist around what is old and broken than to open our hands to receive something new and different. This happens with health care, even if the care we currently receive doesn't make us healthier. We hang on to what we know for all the wrong reasons.

In the next couple of chapters, we'll take a look at some history and attitudes that got us where we are today. Then we'll delve into what *you* can do to bring change to your own health care. Once you see the bigger picture of what's wrong with our health care system, you'll see you don't have to settle for the status quo.

It's time to let go of a broken health care system and venture into real health.

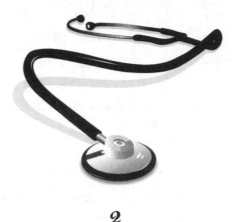

2

It Doesn't Have to Be This Way

Life is about what is working, rather than what is not working.

John Wesley shocked the living daylights out of people.

Not literally. But it was one of his favorite things to do. Public demonstrations of electricity were popular in the mid-eighteenth century. Portable machines using friction electricity astonished crowds by igniting ether or brandy with sparks from people's fingers. John Wesley was infatuated.

Wesley's fascination with shocking people was Benjamin Franklin's fault. Franklin could have killed himself flying a kite with an iron key attached to it during a thunderstorm, but he lived to write pamphlets about electricity. John Wesley studied them. From there it was a short leap to wondering how electricity might be useful in healing physical conditions. Wesley got himself a machine and first shocked himself to treat his own bum leg. Seeing some gradual improvement in his condition, he began offering electric shock to others through the free clinics he operated. Thousands of people tried electric shock. Wesley kept meticulous records and eventually identified thirty-seven disorders he believed responded to the treatment. And in cases where the treatment did not help, it never caused any harm.

Wesley is most famous as a minister and the founder of Methodism, the beginnings of the Methodist Church. What you probably don't know is that Wesley practiced medicine from the age of nineteen until he died. This wasn't just a hobby. He was serious. And it wasn't something he did as a sideline to being a minister because he didn't make enough money evangelizing. It was part and parcel of his ministry and his view of the world, particularly in the health care he offered to the poor. Wesley typically traveled about fifty thousand miles a year around the English countryside on horseback, and he was as interested in healing physical ailments as he was in preaching and promoting Methodist societies. In taking this stance, Wesley joined a long Christian tradition of caring for both body and spirit.

God cares about keeping people well.

The Bible is clear: God's people should care for the poor, the sick, and widows and orphans. Old Testament laws provided for people living on the margins of Israel's society. Ruth, for example, was the widow of an Israelite man and an immigrant caring for her widowed mother-in-law. She made a living gathering grain that harvesters missed because the law of Moses told landowners to leave extra crops for the disadvantaged. The prophet Elijah raised a widow's only son from the dead. Speaking with the authority God gave him, Elisha told Naaman, a military officer, how to treat his skin disease. Jesus healed people practically every time he turned around—the lame, the blind, the dead—and expected his followers to do the same. The early church answered the call and organized itself to care for the poor as well as offer healing.

The book of Acts in the New Testament is full of miraculous healings. But we should not overlook the reality that the early church also expected healing would come through common medical methods. The apostle Paul had a fatherly relationship with Timothy, a young pastor. Paul suggested wine to soothe Timothy's stomach (1 Timothy 5:23), and this would have been nothing surprising at the time. James, a leader of the church in Jerusalem, told believers to call on the elders in times of illness (James 5:14). Today we largely use James's advice to anoint the sick with oil in a ceremonial way, but at the time it was common Greek medical practice to anoint someone and expect it to help. Regardless of what you might think about this advice from your seat in the twenty-first century, the point is the early church felt free to use the best methods doctors of the time offered. Believers had faith that God was able and willing to bring healing through these techniques.

By the fourth century, the Christian faith had spread around the Roman Empire. Church leaders offered both pastoral and medical care. Tradition suggests that Helena, the mother of the emperor Constantine, was the first to open a hospital specifically to care for the poor. More hospitals followed. The ancient world never had a system to care for the sick until Christians offered hospitals. In fact, the church's charity attracted pagans. Julian was a fourth-century Roman emperor who did not have much use for Christians, and thus became known as Julian the Apostate. Yet even Julian saw what happened when Christians cared for the poor. He wrote, "Now we can see what it is that makes those Christians such powerful enemies of our gods. It is the brotherly love which they manifest toward the sick and poor, the thoughtful manner in which they care for the dead, and the purity of their own lives." Unfortunately, when the Roman Empire collapsed in the fifth century, so did this network of health care.

However, the church's healing ministry did not shrivel up completely. During the Middle Ages—centuries of intellectual stagnation and cultural decline—monasteries became centers for health care. Monks cultivated the art of herbal medicine, and when people got sick, they went to see the monks. The Crusades, for all their horror, gave rise to hospices to care for sick pilgrims and crusaders trekking between Europe and Jerusalem. Christians kept medical learning alive while caring for body and spirit.

And then came the Renaissance of Western culture and the Reformation era of church history. False divisions changed fundamental understandings of health care, and we never recovered. These same false divisions still show up in the health care you receive today.

False division 1:
Science and religion stopped playing nice.

Unrest stirred in the dominant body of Christianity in Europe, the Roman Catholic Church. This came to a head in the era of Martin Luther and John Calvin, who "protested" certain theology and practices in the church. The result was "Protestants" who pursued a new understanding of the church. When they broke away from the established church for theological reasons, however, they also cut themselves loose from the system that cared for the sick. Protestants were going to have to find their own feet on the question of a healing ministry, but at the time they were occupied with proving they weren't heretics.

By the eighteenth and nineteenth centuries, scientific knowledge mushroomed. Charles Darwin proposed theories that explained a lot of things without having to bring religion into the discussion. Scientists tugged at the shroud covering the workings of the human body, and a new and improved profession of medicine joined the game. People no longer saw the church as the place to go for care and curing when they were sick. Instead, doctors cared for the body, and it was the church's job to look after the spirit.

Scientists asked questions and found answers, then asked more questions and found more answers. The church did not do very well at keeping up with the conversation. As a branch of science, medicine became a rival to religion. In earlier centuries, people saw new discoveries in medicine as signs of God's work. Now, more and more, medicine was on one path and religious faith was on another path. While scientists and theologians duked it out intellectually, ordinary people found less and less conflict in simply accepting both paths as separate but true.

The union of body and spirit cracked. The fissure split open a gorge, and theologians and scientists could hardly see each other across the expanse. You probably recognize this division because it still rears its head when you get sick. Does faith have any role in making you well, or is it all about science?

False division 2:
Mind and body went their separate ways.

Two thousand years before the Reformation, the Greek philosopher Plato formed the notion that the physical world we can see and touch and taste didn't much matter. True reality was in the soul, which needed to escape from the body. In the seventeenth century, René Descartes picked up the ball and ran with it. Human beings, Descartes said, might be made up of mind and body, but the mind and body are distinct from each other. The body is physical; the mind is not. The mind does not even need the body—the senses— in order to function and figure out what's true. Reason could do the job on its own. The physical and the nonphysical function separately, rather than together. If something broke in the body, science could fix it. What was going on in the nonphysical sphere was irrelevant to questions of the body. At the time, science was making a pretty strong argument that it could understand the physical universe—and certainly the human body—without getting spiritual about it. In this context, Descartes's ideas found a welcome audience. The understanding of physical health was separated from the health of the whole person. Most doctors today still approach health care from the perspective of fixing something broken in the body, rather than looking at the whole person. And most patients go to the doctor looking for a fix for the body without considering that what is happening in their spirits might have something to do with what hurts.

False division 3:
Health ministry gave way to a health industry.

Despite the rift between science and religion, and despite the division of mind and body, medical advances needed practical outlets. The church filled the bill. For instance, the colonies in North America did not have established medical schools to produce doctors for the growing population. As a matter of practicality, pastors and other prominent leaders carried out health care work. A congregational minister might apprentice to a physician, for example, and then become the first source of health care in a rural area. This was true even after the United States formed as an independent nation. Before the Civil War, if you were sick, most likely the first person you saw was the pastor.

In Massachusetts, Cotton Mather was just as zealous about physical health as he was about the spiritual well-being of his late-seventeenth-century congregation. Mather particularly was interested in preventing the epidemics that swept through the population on a regular basis. In 1721 more than half of Boston's ten thousand residents contracted smallpox. Mather's research prompted him to suggest the idea of inoculation and successfully press to see it put into practice. He was a pastor in Boston, but also a significant early figure in American medicine. As a pastor, he argued for the best science could offer and wouldn't settle for less.

Across the ocean, John Wesley held similar views. Keeping

people healthy was essential to his life's ministry, and some medical methods simply needed to stop. Wesley spoke out against antiquated leeching, bleeding, and quicksilver practices. He advocated clean water, fresh air, and exercise—riding a horse would cure anything, in his opinion. Wesley set up dispensaries around England to help the poor, especially coal miners. He aimed his healing ministry at the poor, whom the medical profession neglected because they were not able to pay for services. Wesley tried electric shock for a range of conditions because it was inexpensive and had the potential, in his view, to help people on a large scale for little money.

After the Civil War in the United States, rapid industrial growth pushed a host of social issues to the forefront. Immigrants filled the nation's cities at unprecedented rates. Maybe some of your ancestors arrived during this boon. Labor practices were far from fair. Despite advances in science and medicine, health care remained out of reach for many. In fact, food remained out of reach for many. Churches across denominations came face-to-face with the reality that they could do something. They could take care of the poor and make society better, and perhaps a better society had something to do with God's work in the world. The personalities behind this movement believed everybody should benefit from medical advances, not just the wealthy. Along with Catholic facilities, hospitals sprang up with words like "Baptist," "Methodist," and "Presbyterian" in their names.

People who could afford private doctors continued to call the doctor to their homes in the late nineteenth and early twentieth centuries. Hospitals were places for the poor to go when they had no other option. People with options did not go to the hospital.

And then, around the 1930s, the people of means began to notice something unexpected. People in hospitals got well! In fact, people in hospitals did better than those who stayed home and called the doctor in. This was exciting stuff. Now people from higher economic classes wanted to get involved with hospitals—but they didn't want to pay for them. After all, the Baptists, Methodists, and Presbyterians were doing such a good job paying for everything. People of means essentially said, "The church can keep paying for health care, but we want to help run things and make it better."

This arrangement lasted several decades, but by the 1960s hospitals began to face significant financial challenges. Advances in technology don't come cheap. If you're going to be the best, somebody has to pay for it. The conversation went something like this:

> *Hospital:* Hey, church people, we need money. Remember, you own us, so you should give us the money.
> *Church:* Sorry, but we have our own problems. Find the money yourself.
> *Hospital:* Okay, we'll hire a hospital administrator. It can be a new kind of job. We'll pay somebody to figure out this mess.
> *Church:* Yeah, whatever, if you think that's best. We're not giving you more money.

And then—Medicare and Medicaid! Starting in 1965, federal money was poured into the funding of hospitals. The arrival of these government programs triggered the spending of billions of dollars on developing a hospital system for the poor and elderly. Hospitals found a way to actually make money by taking care of sick people. Now medicine was big business. Across the country, in city after city, health care became the largest employer category. People carried little cards that guaranteed someone else would pay the hospital. The more services the hospital provided, the more money someone paid them. About twenty years later, the church thought, *Something is wrong with this picture*, and here's how the conversation went:

Church: Hey, hospital people, our name is on the sign. How come we don't get any of the money?

Hospital: You snooze, you lose. We did it without you after all. We're keeping the money.

Church: But our name is on the sign.

Hospital: We dare you to do something about it.

A firewall went up between churches and the hospitals they opened in the first place. It didn't make sense any longer for churches to own hospitals since they didn't make the decisions and they didn't benefit financially from the business. Denominations began to sell the hospitals they had opened decades earlier to for-profit companies. Now the church had nothing to do with running hospitals. The signs still said "Baptist," "Methodist," or "Presbyterian," but that was largely for historical purposes. Even now, decades later, you may go to a hospital that has a church-sounding word buried somewhere in the name that resulted from mergers and not think much of it. You're there because they have the technology or specialist you need and the hospital is in your insurance plan. But it was the church that started the ball rolling long before anyone figured out how to turn a profit from caring for people who are sick.

In the course of a hundred years, hospitals shifted from providing health care for the poor to being profitable. Despite the advances of the twentieth century, by 2000, the poor once again were left outside the health care system.

Let's go back to the right questions.

What happened to understanding the healing ministry of the church—from the healing miracles in the Bible to John Wesley's electric shock machine to hospitals that did not require a magic card?

Multiple times in history, the church has answered the call to offer cure and caring as God's presence in the world. However, the rift between science and religion, the philosophic separation of the mind from the body, and a business model for health care added up to a battle the church chose not to fight. The church went from being the movers and shakers in health care to observers standing on the sidelines.

The question now is, does it have to be this way? Do we have to settle for this? My answer is no. I don't think the system is working particularly well. If it were, we wouldn't be in the mess we're in when it comes to health care. You may not be able to go back and change history, but you can learn from it. What does *health* mean to you? What is the spiritual element of your life that affects your wellness? What can you do to care for your own health and be a healing presence in the lives of people around you? Life is about what is working, rather than what is *not* working. Let's put things in their proper places and rediscover health care you can live with.

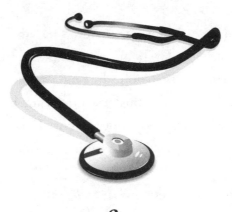

3

Health Care Rides the Technology Wave

We have an unholy love affair with technology.

Aziz's Pakistani accent was so thick I could barely understand him, but I could see he was distressed. "I feel like I am a ticking time bomb," he said. Aziz needed a procedure people undergo every day. His carotid artery, which supplies blood flow to the brain, was clogged with plaque. Without the surgery, Aziz might have a stroke. He understood he needed the procedure, and a surgeon was available to perform it.

Only one problem. Aziz owed money to the surgeon's medical practice. The business manager told him he was welcome to return and schedule the surgery once he cleared up his account from a previous procedure.

An unholy love affair with technology led to this situation and others like it that happen every day. Technology and business have hijacked health care. Aziz is a victim of the rift between science and religion that made it so easy for the church to step out of a healing ministry and leave it to science to develop a healing business in its place.

The cost of insurance.

The cost of seeing doctors.

The cost of medications.

The cost of a hospital stay.

The cost of an operation.

Conversation about health care seems to be more about cost than about health. In the twenty-first century it's difficult to talk about health care and not talk about technology. A big part of why health care is so expensive involves the price of technology. We live in an age when last year's new electronic gadget is out of date. But what does that have to do with making you healthier? Let's step back for a moment and look at how technology has shaped our health care system. Then we might be able to sort out its rightful place as we move forward to healthier lives.

Technology has leveled off.

Think back a hundred years. Medical technology was a far cry from what it is today. No MRIs. No CT scans. No bypass surgery. No organ transplants. No penicillin or other antibiotics. No pacemakers. No vaccines for polio or measles or influenza. No specialized practices. The list could go on and on. Chances are that every person you know has benefited from technology that did not exist a hundred years ago, or even fifty years ago. When the twentieth century opened, we were at the bottom of the chart, and few people imagined what the century would bring to the world of health care. While doctors' understanding of the human body was growing by leaps and bounds, when things went wrong, they still had few treatments to offer patients other than a sympathetic bedside manner and a handful of pharmaceuticals. Some treatments were based more on folklore than science.

New medical technology of the twentieth century remarkably improved our ability to treat disease and improve quality of life.

With the help of technology, we figured out how to fix a lot of things that go wrong in the human body. Even relatively small advances in technology yielded wide benefits to many people. People got healthier and generally lived longer. Just the discovery of penicillin alone revolutionized treatment for many conditions and saved untold lives. Today simple medications can control conditions that once were a death sentence, and if medications are not enough, dramatic procedures are more common and safer than ever. We believe that no matter what the situation, technology can solve the problem. Too many of us have the attitude that it doesn't matter how I've lived my life, what I eat, how many cigarettes I smoke, how long I sit on the couch. Technology can fix what happens even when I persist in unhealthy habits. I can go to the doctor, and the doctor will know how to fix the problem. And if a little technology is good, imagine what we could do with a lot of technology!

But we are not at the bottom of the technology chart anymore. We're at the top of the chart. The line that used to rise dramatically, recording the advances of technology, has leveled off. It's moving, more or less, straight across the top of the chart until it falls off the page.

We're top-heavy with technology when it comes to health care. The medical community has become like restless teenagers who insist on having the newest electronic gadget. An entire economy swirls around buying the latest technology, and this includes the way doctors practice medicine. In the United States we take pride in the fact that more than thirty cities each have more MRI scanners than all of Canada. And at each facility with an MRI machine, physicians and marketers pressure for the latest and greatest, the new and improved version, the one with the best "wow" factor. A laboratory or research company develops it. A marketing and sales staff makes sure physicians know about it. Radiologists, for instance, see that the new MRI gives a prettier, slightly more detailed picture of the body, so they must have this new version.

Technology just knocked over the first business domino.

Because the radiologists are enamored by the new MRI machine, they pressure the hospital to invest in one. Hospital administrators hem and haw about the cost, but eventually they cave in and buy it because they want to claim to be the best. That means having top-of-the-line equipment and attracting premier specialists. They can't risk patients or doctors going to another hospital that has a machine they don't have. That's plain bad for business.

Insurance companies cave in and agree to pay for procedures using this new equipment because savvy corporate executives have heard about it. These industry leaders want to know where to go for the latest technology, and if one insurance company won't give it to them, another will. The cost of this new technology is astronomical, but the bottom line is doctors and hospitals can't stay in business without keeping up.

Our thirst for new health care technology is irrational. Here's why: It doesn't make you better.

The cost of health care is rising out of control in part because of this thirst for new technology. Each newest or latest version is going to cost a fortune to develop and introduce. Nobody disputes that. Thousands of jobs depend on developing, selling, buying, and delivering new technology. But because we're already at the top of the chart, ready to tip off the page, the next version is going to be only slightly better than the one before, or it might be simply a more convenient redesign of the same features and elements. In the United States, we claim to have the best health care system in the world. This is not because our people generally are healthier—they aren't—but because we have more technology than any other country, and more people have access to it.

We have reached a point where expectations are completely unrealistic. A new MRI machine may improve the quality of the image of the human body, but for the most part it does not improve the quality of care you receive. In fact, the new picture probably won't change your doctor's plan for how to take care of you at all.

Pills are poison.

So forget the expensive machines. The state of prescription medications follows the same pattern.

The Federal Drug Administration rates new drugs based on whether they represent significant improvement over the drugs already available. In the last twenty years, the FDA classified the overwhelming majority of new drugs as "me too" drugs. They looked just like something already in use as a generic. Perhaps developers changed a molecule or two to be able to present the chemical combination as a new product. In recent decades, the FDA has rated not more than a handful of drugs as true improvements. Yet we see drugs with catchy new names advertised on television every day. People go into a doctor's office convinced they need a particular medication, but the ads are aimed even more directly at physicians. Doctors will say the advertisements don't affect them, but the ads are incredibly effective. And they don't just show up in television commercials; they also appear in the professional literature physicians read—mailed to them for free.

The medications we shake out of prescription or over-the-counter bottles essentially act the way poisons act. They invade the body to prevent it from doing something the body is trying to do naturally. That's how a poison works—it stops a natural process from happening. In general, this is the way medications work. People believe drugs cure disease, but they don't. Rather, they interfere with a process gone wrong so your body's own immune system can kick in and take over. Antibiotics don't kill bacteria, for instance. Your immune system does the job because the antibiotic helps your system work faster and more effectively. And a lot of minor illnesses improve without medications. A patient once called me at two in the morning, distressed that a colleague refused to give her antibiotics for her sore throat the previous day. She was convinced she needed medicine, when what she really needed was patience for a couple of days—and perhaps some honey in her tea. Every doctor has stories like that.

The truth is most pills don't work very well. Medications have limited efficiency and long lists of side effects. If pills did everything they promised on television, doctors would be killing people right and left. If pills actually did their job and influenced the body's systems as vigorously as the television commercials claim, you'd be in trouble every time you took a pill.

We need a new chart.

I am not arguing that we should halt the technological advance of American medicine. I myself benefit from a prosthetic hip that has relieved years of pain. Yet, after practicing medicine for twenty-five years, I recognize that new technology does not automatically improve the patient's health, and we need to stop thinking it does. Sometimes it is hard to justify the cost a facility charges for using this technology when, going in, doctors know the latest version of technology is not going to result in a change in the plan for treating the patient.

My point is this: We no longer see the huge forward leaps of medical technology we saw fifty or a hundred years ago, when large portions of the population benefited. The changes in technology we see now are tweaks and adjustments compared to the discoveries and inventions of the past century. Yet we continue to pour vast amounts of money into a system that is not making people healthier. We make these advances in technology because we can—scientifically—and because doing so supports a major sector of our economy. A system that leads to improved health of Americans would impact the pocketbooks of almost everyone working in health care. A healthier population means fewer pills, fewer tests, and ultimately, fewer dollars spent on technology and pharmaceuticals. In the process of creating an industry based on technology, we lose sight of the fact that health care is supposed to be about health.

So what system would make people healthier?

Understanding what it means to be well—body and spirit. And developing behaviors and lifestyles that focus on what works, not on what is broken. That's the essence of prevention.

Technology absorbs the time, talent, and resources we need for keeping us healthy—it generally isn't needed until we break. Take childhood obesity as an example. It's frequently in the news, and it should be. We are raising a generation of kids who go home from school, sit on the couch, play on the Xbox, and eat junk food. These obese children *will* be adults who have hypertension, diabetes, heart attacks, and trouble finding employment and fitting into society. But we have to do more than talk about it and look at pictures of sedentary children eating processed food. If we dedicate resources to fighting obesity through preventing it in the first place, we can make a far greater difference in the health of a generation than will ever come from developing a next-generation MRI or new drugs for erectile dysfunction. Because of our love affair with technology, we are failing to give children hope for their futures. While we debate how to give them access to technology in the event that their bodies break down—and they will—we overlook giving them the love and joy and self-understanding essential to real health of the whole person.

While we're at the top of the chart when it comes to technology, we're at the bottom of the chart when it comes to prevention. We have not even begun to explore the widespread benefit that could come from aiming resources at keeping people well in the first place. We've invested only a miniscule amount in answering questions about what prevention should look like because there is no financial incentive to do so. Focusing exclusively on the cost of health care (or more accurately, the way we spend money on health care) prevents us from achieving true health care reform.

The heart of a health care system that focuses on keeping you well—preventing bodily breakdowns—requires a return to the belief that caring for people's health is a helping profession, not big business. True health care reform would create incentives for prevention and focus on keeping people healthy so they need less technology, rather than presenting access to technology as the answer to every bad habit. Research would shift away from technology and drugs to early treatment of disease through primary care. We need a system that makes people healthier and happier—full of joy and love. That's a huge corner to turn at this point in time.

Churches—and individual Christians—can get back in the game by reclaiming their own understanding of wellness and care that promotes health for themselves and their communities. You don't have to buy into the belief that technology is the answer to everything. It's not. You can value what technology brings to your health without getting sucked into thinking that technology is the heart of health care. It's not. Individual choices make a difference. *Your* choices make a difference in your health. You can turn the discussion away from questions of costs and systems to questions that connect you to God in the way God means for you to be connected. Then you can truly begin to care for your health.

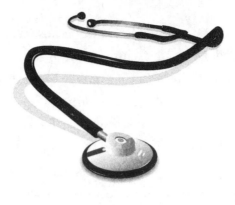

4

Plato Was Wrong

"We relate to God from the neck up." Wrong!

Marcia was convinced she had cancer. At thirty-two years of age, her body hurt from head to toe, and she was giving me every detail. In the middle of her litany, I stopped her to ask, "Why did you move to Memphis?"

She hesitated then said, "I had to get away. My husband is getting out of jail tomorrow."

"So why was he in jail?"

"For abusing me and my children."

"Do you think he will come after you now?"

Marcia looked at the floor. "He might."

She came in to tell me about her fear of cancer, but it seemed to me that the cancer was in her relationship with this abusive man. Most physicians hear a complaint of a specific symptom and quickly focus on possible physical causes. I've learned to bring the non-physical into the conversation fairly early. Spiritual or relational strain may be the real reason a patient comes to see me. Plato was wrong. Descartes was wrong. We can't separate body from spirit.

What is the real me?

The real you is body and spirit, together and inseparable. Human beings are not one part body and one part spirit. We are *body-and-spirit*. Philosophers like Plato and Descartes want us to believe we can dissect ourselves into the physical part and the nonphysical part, and the two don't have anything to do with each other. In fact, some would argue we may do whatever we want with our bodies because the physical life has nothing to do with true existence in the spirit.

That couldn't be further from the truth. From a biblical point of view, we cannot separate body and spirit. God simply never meant for that to happen. God formed Adam from the dust of the earth and breathed into him the breath of life, and "the man became a living being" (Genesis 2:7). God did not create a body and as an afterthought add a spirit. God did not create a spirit and then decide it would be more practical to house it in a body. From the moment of creation, humans were body-and-spirit. God's breath of life became intimately mixed with clay from the ground, and from that point on, body-and-spirit were inseparable.

God created human beings to exist in a relationship with God. The lush Garden of Eden, God's creation, was a very physical setting, and God put Adam and Eve there—and God was there, too. God walked in the garden in the cool of the day and spoke to Adam and Eve (Genesis 3:8). God did not simply create spirits to swirl around and perhaps mix with God's Spirit. Rather, God created body-and-spirit beings, put them in a physical place, and met them there. The creation story tells us that our physical existence—our body—is a gift from God.

We know God with our bodies.

The idea that we relate to God from the neck up—without our whole bodies—is nonsense. In the Old Testament, we read many examples of a bodily, physical expression of our relationship with God. David, the greatest king of Israel, "danced before the LORD with all his might" (2 Samuel 6:14). And why did David dance? Not just because he liked the way it felt. He danced to celebrate before the Lord when Israel defeated the enemy Philistines (2 Samuel 6:21). The ark of the Lord—the very presence of God among the people of God—returned to Jerusalem after the battle, and David let loose to worship the Lord by dancing with all his might. David was a terribly flawed individual in many ways, but he understood that he lived in relationship to God in every way. He did not limit himself to quiet prayers; he showed enormous physical exuberance for God.

The Psalms of the Old Testament give us vivid pictures of our inseparable body-and-spirit need for God. Notice the link between spiritual themes and physical imagery in these verses:

> Be merciful to me, O LORD, for I am in distress;
>> my eyes grow weak with sorrow,
>> my soul and my body with grief. (Psalm 31:9)

> O God, you are my God,
>> earnestly I seek you;
> my soul thirsts for you,
>> my body longs for you
> in a dry and weary land
>> where there is no water. (Psalm 63:1)

> When I was in distress, I sought the Lord;
>> at night I stretched out untiring hands
>> and my soul refused to be comforted.
> I remembered you, O God, and I groaned;
>> I mused, and my spirit grew faint. (Psalm 77:2–3)

The psalmist did not relate to God from the neck up. His whole being, body-and-spirit, was involved. The Psalms tell us to lift our eyes to God (121:1–2), use our voices to cry to God (116:1), lift our hands (134:2), sing and make all kinds of music (147:7; 150:3–4). On one occasion when God's people celebrated the action of God, the psalmist said, "Our mouths were filled with laughter, our tongues with songs of joy" (126:2). Sensory, physical imagery runs rampant in the Psalms because God created the body and declared it good, and because we relate to God as whole beings, body-and-spirit.

Ezekiel is another great Old Testament example that the body is no accident or secondary creation. A prophet during a difficult time in the history of God's people, Ezekiel had some bizarre experiences. One was a vision of a valley cluttered with dry bones. God led Ezekiel back and forth among the bones and asked, "Can these bones live?" Then God told Ezekiel to say to the bones, "I will make breath enter you, and you will come to life" (Ezekiel 37:3, 5). Ezekiel did as he was told and the bones came to life—a vast army standing in the valley. God gave a very physical picture—a bodily picture—of assurance that God was active in what was happening among the people of God.

Using a body to communicate with God's people made sense because God created the union of body-and-spirit in the first place and always intended that we respond with body-and-spirit.

God redeems all of you.

By the time New Testament writers lived and worked, clearly a separation of body and spirit had invaded the thinking of the culture. By then, Plato had come on the scene with his notion that the physical could be separated from the nonphysical. In Plato's view, the world we experience through our senses somehow is defective, so all that matters is the nonphysical world. In fact, Plato said, the soul does not even need the body to exist.

The apostle Paul, who shaped so much of Christian thought with his letters to churches, ranted and raved against this division. First-century Christians in various cities were sucked into thinking they could do whatever they wanted with their bodies because God had already given them salvation for their souls. This couldn't be further from the truth. We can well imagine the scribe—taking Paul's dictation and scribbling on parchment—could hardly keep up with the torrent of words. Salvation of the soul is no excuse for loose morality of the body, especially when it comes to sexual relationships (1 Corinthians 6:13). Salvation of the soul is no excuse for side-stepping the truth that God wants all of you, body-and-spirit, as a living sacrifice (Romans 12:1). Salvation of the soul is no excuse for believing one thing with the mind and doing another thing with the body (Ephesians 4:4). In fact, Paul takes great pains to explain that God redeems not just our souls, but all of creation—including our physical bodies (Romans 8:22–23).

John was one of Jesus' closest friends. Decades after the three intense years he spent with Jesus, John wrote to Christians about the nitty-gritty of living in the world and in relationships. The same sort of false teachers Paul ranted against were active in the faith communities John wrote to. John's approach is direct: Live your bodily life in a way that shows you belong to God. Separating faith from action is not an option because we don't exist in two spheres. John wrote with firm teaching on the subject in the letter of 1 John. But he also wrote with a tender heart in 3 John. To his friend Gaius he said, "I pray that you may enjoy good health and that all may go well with you, even as your soul is getting along well" (3 John 2).

Health means wellness in body-and-spirit.

Not body or spirit, separate.

Not body and spirit, separate but somehow connected.

Body-and-spirit. Together. One whole person.

Despite Plato, despite Descartes, despite science, despite technology, the fact remains that the real you is body-and-spirit. What God loves is you, body-and-spirit. God invites you into a relationship in body-and-spirit. What happens in your body is not separate from what happens in your spirit. We, whole human beings, know God through our bodies as well as our spirits, and even when we fail, God comes to us in our physical experience. We know ourselves most fully when we know ourselves in relation to God as whole beings, body-and-spirit.

If you want real health, you have to start with the real you. Understanding that God cares about your body may be a new starting point for you, but it is the right starting point. You honor God when you care for your body. The health care system may be a mess, but you don't have to be. Reclaiming your health begins with reclaiming God's view of the real you.

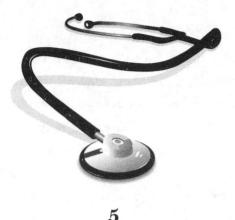

5

Cherish Being Human

*The enfleshing of Jesus says something of what
God thinks of being human.*

By the time I saw Leonida for the first time, she had been to the walk-in clinic of the Church Health Center on several occasions because of stomach pain. She was back again to hear the results of an ultrasound to try to ferret out the source of the pain, because her stomach still hurt.

An older woman from one of the local churches was with Leonida. She held Leonida's daughter, Anna Paula. I quickly learned that this Brazilian family was in Memphis because Anna Paula had a terrible disease called osteopetrosis, which leads to major deformity of the skeletal system. For most of her eight years, Anna Paula had been a patient at St. Jude Children's Research Hospital. The family was in the United States. on a medical visa, which meant they could not work. They scrimped by for seven years, but the strain was getting to all of them, and Anna Paula was not getting better. In fact, she recently had gone blind and lost her teeth because of the progression of the disease and could walk only with great difficulty.

Leonida's test results were normal. I hoped that would encourage her, but I could see in her face that she knew the pain in her stomach was nothing medicine would chase away. Body and spirit were bound together in the experience of her daughter's illness.

When the body fails us, it's tempting to think maybe Plato was right and we should seek to separate the soul from the body so the soul can go off to someplace far away from this planet and live eternally without the confinement and disappointments of a body.

But that's Plato and not Jesus. Jesus gives us quite another picture of being human and the challenge to cherish the nature of being human.

What does it mean to be human?

The enfleshing of Jesus, God's own Son, says something of what God thinks of being human. God created the physical world and called it "good." God created human beings and said, "*very* good." Then God gave Jesus human birth, human flesh, human experience.

Jesus was human.

Jesus slept when he was tired, walked everywhere he went, sat on hillsides, anticipated questions, told stories, paid taxes, stroked the heads of children, loved his own mother, made his siblings wait, experienced temptation, cried over the death of a close friend, acted with compassion, enjoyed good meals, debated with cultural leaders, talked to people he "should have known better" than to be seen with, pointed out the errors of his best friends, washed dirty feet.

Jesus was human.

Nothing about human existence surprises Jesus, because he's been in our shoes. He lived life within the confines and disappointments of a body. Four different writers filled their accounts of Jesus' life with details and gave us the Gospels of Matthew, Mark, Luke, and John at the beginning of the New Testament. John, one of Jesus' closest friends, writes in a more theological style than the others, but even his starting point is that Jesus took on flesh. The Word of God—God's own Son—became human and lived a human life among other humans. While he lived on earth, Jesus was not just a spiritual being hiding in a physical body. He was flesh and blood. He was human. God created humanity, including the body, and did not hesitate to send Jesus to experience what we experience. That tells us something about what God thinks of the human body.

"What about the miracles?" you might be asking right about now. "What about the crucifixion? Jesus' life was about more than eating, sleeping, and going to parties."

Yes. Exactly.

Jesus lived a life of faith connected to God. He never drifted away from this anchor. Being human and living in a human body did not separate Jesus from God. Being human put Jesus right where God wanted him to be, to do the work God wanted him to do. Jesus' ministry included preaching to the crowds, teaching his followers, and healing people whose bodies failed them—in order to show God's power at work. He healed lame people, deaf people, blind people, leprous people, demon-possessed people, even dead people. Jesus cared about bodies because he cared about the whole person in relationship to God. Living a life of faith in the body is not just for Jesus. God wants this for all of us. This is the core of being human.

God works in the body-and-spirit.

Jesus' disciples knew body and spirit had something to do with each other, but they didn't quite get the relationship right. They saw a man who had been born blind, and they asked Jesus, "Who sinned, this man or his parents?" (John 9:2). They were sure the man was physically blind because of a spiritual offense against God. Jesus' answer was that nobody's sin caused the blindness. Then Jesus spat in the dirt, mixed up some mud, smeared it on the man's eyes, and told him to go wash his face. After the man washed, he could see.

This stirred up quite a bit of controversy. Neighbors tried to convince themselves the man wasn't the same guy they walked past every day. Religious leaders demanded to know how he received his sight—then refused to believe his story. They asked his parents what happened, and his parents said, "Ask him yourself." So the leaders asked the man again. By now he was losing patience and started to talk back, so they threw him out, still not believing someone who sinned as much as he had could be healed.

This story in John 9 is more about spiritual blindness than physical blindness. The religious leaders refused to open their eyes and see the truth—that God was at work. Jesus cared enough about the man's blindness to do something about it, and in the process, he pointed to the power of God in the man's life. In healing a physical problem, Jesus also cleared away spiritual blindness so the man could see God more clearly. The religious leaders of the time, trapped in their own spiritual blindness, could not get their heads around the fact that God might work in a way they did not expect.

We should not presume that what goes wrong in the body is a result of someone's sin, though some behaviors have natural consequences that lead to illness. God works in the body— miraculously or through the gift of knowledge and medicine— because God does not see us as divided between body and spirit, but as whole individuals who need divine grace in our lives.

God's grace comes to us in physical, visceral ways. The gospel writers give us gruesome detail of the physical experience of Jesus sacrificing himself so that we can have peace with God. Soldiers slammed nails through his hands and feet, ripping through skin, tendon, muscle, and bone. They smashed a crown of thorns into his head. They stabbed a spear into his side and bodily fluids poured out. Jesus died on that rugged cross. Jesus did not simply think in his mind, *I'll save these humans who lost their way,* and then suddenly everything was okay. He agonized about the experience so profoundly that he was sweating blood and praying for a way out. But he went through with it, suffering in his body because humans are created body-and-spirit.

Three days later, God raised Jesus from the dead in his body. The resurrection was not only spiritual; it was physical. The tomb was empty because the body was no longer dead. Hundreds of people saw Jesus. He spoke to his disciples. He invited Thomas to touch him. He made a fire and cooked breakfast on the beach. He took a walk with Peter for a private conversation. All of this was bodily. New Testament writers herald that we, too, will experience resurrection at the end of time. We may not know all the details of how the body will be transformed or when exactly this will happen, but we know that we will have bodies going into eternity with God. God does not say, "I made a mistake with this body business. Let's just worry about the spirit." Over and over, the Bible tells us God values the body and comes to us in our experience with the body.

Live life to the full.

Our bodies disappoint us. We can have no doubt about that. Even apart from dangerous behaviors or accidents, bodies break. They grow cells they should not grow. Organs fail. Sometimes bodies hurt and we don't ever know why. We live with chronic illness, even suffering that seems as though it should be unbearable. Loved ones die while we hold their hands and cool their foreheads and give them one last kiss.

But none of this means that the body is not at the heart of how we know God. Jesus lived in connection to God without separating body from spirit. He understood that his life had purpose and meaning—precisely through his physical experience, not in spite of it. The apostle Paul calls Jesus' death "God's abundant provision of grace" (Romans 5:17). Jesus himself said he came so we can "have life, and have it to the full" (John 10:10).

Jesus brings life to body-and-spirit. God means for us to cherish the nature of being human in body-and-spirit. Through it all we are connected to God, who calls us to live a life of faith in and through the body, just as Jesus did. When John Wesley shocked people, it was because he saw wellness of the body as part of how we respond to God's call on our lives. Rather than pushing the body aside in your understanding of what it means to live a full life, embrace it. See from Jesus' example what it means to be human and intimately connected to God.

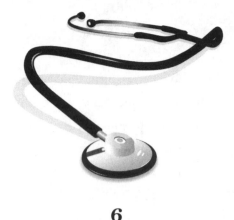

6

The Body Brings Us Together

*Jesus gave us enough examples of mercy to
challenge us for a lifetime.*

I was livid.

In the early days of the Church Health Center, I worried about people taking advantage of our low-cost services. Would people come in and not tell the truth about their financial resources? Since we operated on the goodness of people's gifts, I felt an obligation to make sure we were good stewards of the gifts. That included making sure people who came through our doors did not abuse our system. So I used to do parking lot patrol. At random intervals, I wandered through the parking lot and inspected the cars. If I saw a car that looked like the driver was doing pretty well financially, I would find out who drove it.

One day I discovered a Jaguar.

I stormed through the clinic until I discovered the driver and demanded to know why someone who could afford to drive a Jaguar came to the Church Health Center. It turned out to be an older guy who worked for the Jaguar dealership in some low-level capacity.

That day his own heap of junk wouldn't start, so his boss gave him the keys to his personal vehicle—a Jag—so the patient wouldn't miss his appointment with the doctor.

I ceased the parking lot patrols. Do some people take advantage of us? Quite likely. But we don't always know the whole story, and jumping to conclusions because we're trying to protect ourselves actually can get in the way of providing health care to the poor.

And protecting ourselves is not what the church is about.

You are the body of Christ.

We are body-and-spirit, created and loved by God, and our bodies are a gift from God. We are connected to God by our bodies, not only our spirits. God values the body enough to send Jesus into a fully human existence and to use the bodily experience of Jesus as the way to bring humans into relationship with God. The apostle Paul understood the powerful imagery of the body enough to use it as the primary picture of God's people in the world.

Christians in first-century Corinth squabbled—a lot, apparently. They quarreled about allegiance to leaders. They argued about the essence of the gospel message. They debated the pros and cons of participating in the culture around them. They jockeyed to get the "best" gifts for ministry—worship and Christian living. That one congregation is a compelling argument that nothing much is new in the church. Paul's answer is just as enduring: Remember, above all things, you are the body of Christ. One Spirit baptizes believers into one body.

"You are the body of Christ."

That should make us pause. We are the hands and feet, the eyes and ears of Jesus. We are the body of Jesus that the world sees. A body is a visible, palpable, physical presence. If we are the body of Christ, shouldn't we be doing what Jesus did?

Care about what Jesus cared about.

I was at a conference at the Carter Center in Atlanta, Georgia, and heard former president Jimmy Carter speak. He personally had gone through the Gospels and tallied the number of verses related to healing. By his count, fully one-third of the gospel narratives involve healing. Jesus teaches, preaches, and heals. Healing is a third of his ministry, so we can't ignore it. Take the Gospel of Luke and set it beside the book of Acts, which Luke also wrote, and the theme is clear. If you want to be a follower of Jesus, then you must take to heart the teachings of Jesus, and you must do what Jesus did.

In Luke 10, we read the story of Jesus sending seventy of his followers out in pairs. Jesus sent followers out to announce that the kingdom of God—God's sovereign rule—is here and now. Jesus gave specific instructions for how his followers should respond if people received them in peace and what to do if they met hostility. At the heart of those specific, explicit instructions, Jesus said, "Heal the sick who are there and tell them, 'The kingdom of God is near you'" (Luke 10:9). Jesus was not going along on this particular trek; he was sending his followers—with specific instructions to heal as part of their announcement of the kingdom. Clearly he expected them to heal. He expected them to do as they saw him do over and over again. They should expect to see God's kingdom power working through their actions. And when the seventy followers returned, they said, "Lord, even the demons submit to us in your name" (Luke 10:17). They perhaps were astonished at their own message of the kingdom.

Luke is the only one of the gospel writers to tell this story, and he continues his theme in the book of Acts. Peter and Paul, the towering leaders of the early church, preached and taught, but they also healed. Luke recounts nineteen different healing stories in Acts, and likely these were only the highlights. Luke points out more than once that the apostles did "many wonders and miraculous signs" among the people (Acts 2:43; 5:12; 14:3; 19:11). Both Peter and Paul healed people who had never been able to walk. Paul himself received a healing miracle. When he encountered Christ for the first time on the road to Damascus, the experience left him blind. God sent a Christian named Ananias to find Paul and heal him. God demonstrated healing through Paul's ministry so consistently that people brought handkerchiefs and aprons for him to touch and took them back to cure their sick loved ones (Acts 19:12). Even as a Roman prisoner shipwrecked after a bad storm because someone made a stubborn sailing decision, Paul had a healing ministry to strangers on an island (Acts 28:8–9).

Peter and Paul even have resurrection stories. When a woman named Tabitha died and Peter was staying in a nearby town, the Christians went to fetch him. Clearly these believers expected healing was possible even in the face of death. They did not merely report Tabitha's demise. They said, "Please come at once!" (Acts 9:38). Peter didn't shrug them off and say there was nothing he could do now that Tabitha was dead. He went with them to see what healing God might choose to do. When Peter arrived to a mass of mourners crying and remembering Tabitha's life, he did not merely say, "She lived a good life." He dedicated himself to the task of bringing healing. He went upstairs to the room where Tabitha died and where her body still lay, and there he got down on his knees and prayed. Then he said, "Tabitha, get up." And she opened her eyes, saw Peter, and sat up. Peter escorted her back downstairs, a talking and walking announcement of the kingdom of God.

Paul knew a captive audience when he saw one. One Sunday in Troas, the Christians gathered to worship, and Paul was the featured speaker. Since he planned to leave the next day, he couldn't say, "We'll pick this up next week." Instead, he talked all day and all the way up to midnight. A young man named Eutychus sat in an open third-story window. As much as he might have thought he wanted to hear Paul teach, Eutychus got tired and dropped into a sound sleep—and then plummeted to the ground from that third-story window. No doubt Paul lost some of his audience as they rushed to see what happened. In fact, Paul himself went downstairs. Not surprisingly, Eutychus was dead. But Paul threw himself on him and said, "Don't be alarmed. He's alive!" (Acts 20:10). And he was.

I'm not saying every Christian will go around performing miracles and raising the dead; that's up to God. But I am saying Jesus calls all who follow him to demonstrate the same priority of healing of the whole person, body-and-spirit, that he showed. He asks us to care about what he cares about—wellness and wholeness. Healing that flows through personal care, preventive activities, medical methods, and technology announces that the kingdom of God is here. We cannot separate healing from the gospel message. If we're going to do what Jesus did, and as his first-century followers did, we must find some way to be involved in a ministry of healing. The church—the body of Christ—must show the here-and-now nature of the kingdom of God through healing.

Mercy is compassion in action.

Jesus said, "Blessed are the merciful, for they will be shown mercy" (Matthew 5:7). Our actions should reflect God and the relationship we have with God because of mercy. And what is mercy but compassion in action?

Jesus was willing to care for Peter's mother-in-law when she was lying in bed with a fever. What a great thing to do for your friend.

A Roman military officer came to Jesus and asked for help for his servant who was suffering with a serious illness. The Jews were not particularly fond of Roman rule. No one would have faulted Jesus for walking away. Instead, he embraced the need of the servant—and the officer's respect for Jesus' authority—and healed the servant.

When an expert in the Jewish law tried to entice Jesus into

debate, Jesus pointed him back to the law the man already knew: Love God, love your neighbor. But the expert in the law did what experts do and looked for the loophole. "Who is my neighbor?" In other words, "Who do I really have to be responsible for? And who can I just ignore?"

At this point, Jesus changed the tone of the debate and told a story. A man traveling on the steep and dangerous road between Jerusalem and Jericho fell into the hands of bandits who beat him senseless and left him to die. Religious leaders followed the letter of the law, and rather than risk being temporarily "unclean" by touching a body that might be dead, they crossed to the other side of the road. The traveler who eventually stopped was a Samaritan. The Jews and the Samaritans had nothing good to say about each other and generally went out of their way to avoid each other. Yet this was the traveler who stopped, inconvenienced himself, spent money, and made a commitment to restore health to the Jewish traveler. "Who was the neighbor?" Jesus asked.

The answer was obvious, even to the expert.

Our neighbors are all around us.

The call to mercy is not to figure out the reasonable limits of mercy, but to embrace its unlimited nature. Jesus tells us to put compassion in action, even if it costs us something.

Romero usually held two jobs to keep the bills paid and care for his wife and four children. He was no slacker. But sometimes he had to choose between taking care of his family by working odd jobs at night and taking care of his diabetes and hypertension. Over the years, both diseases weakened his kidneys, and now he needed dialysis. Soon. Under federal law, the government must pay for this treatment. But not for Romero. Although he had lived and worked in the United States for twenty years, he was not a citizen, so the law didn't cover him. He faced the choice of continuing to work and care for his family as long as he could, or leaving his four children, all U.S. citizens, to return to Mexico—where he might or might not receive dialysis.

How does the body of Christ pour out healing mercy for someone like Romero?

Silvia came to me with hepatitis A when she was seventeen. She grew up in Atlanta with her brother, her mother, and her mother's boyfriend. Over the years both the brother and the boyfriend sexually abused her. When she was sixteen, her grandmother found out and petitioned for custody. But Silvia's grandmother only wanted the state check that came with custody. She paid little attention to Silvia. Eventually Silvia ran away, lived on her own, and found her way to Memphis. Three weeks before she came to the Church Health Center, Silvia met Eric and soon moved in with him and his mother, the woman who brought her to see me when she became ill.

How does the body of Christ pour out healing mercy for someone like Silvia?

Amanda came to me saying she believed she had lupus, a form of arthritis that develops because a person's own antibodies start attacking body parts as though they are foreign. She may very well have had lupus, but her family situation was equally distressing. Two years earlier she had married a Serbian man with an extreme authoritarian attitude. He soon brought multiple family members to the United States to live with them. Amanda worked all day and came home to cook for a family she did not know, who did not speak English, and for whom she gave up her bed.

How does the body of Christ pour out healing mercy for someone like Amanda?

God's mercy for us is unlimited. God poured out rich mercy in sending Jesus to share our flesh. God poured out rich mercy in giving the Holy Spirit to keep us connected to God. When we least deserve it, God pours out mercy on us out of love for us, body-and-spirit. Jesus gave us enough examples of mercy—compassion in action—to challenge us for a lifetime. Mercy springs up throughout the New Testament, bursting into view just when we think we are free of its demands.

Find your healing ministry.

What does a healing ministry look like in today's world? At the Church Health Center, we're trying to figure that out every day. Many of our staff come to us precisely because they're trying to figure it out in their own lives. Ann, an attorney, always struggled with how she could serve the poor. She just did not see that her arsenal of gifts and temperament equipped her for face-to-face approaches, but she wanted to do something meaningful. The Church Health Center opened an avenue for her to work in a way she believes makes a difference. Kevin's wife says he works at Disneyland, because she sees the joy he takes in our ministry's work. At the Church Health Center, Jenny sees how faith can be a connector rather than a divider. Mike sees our work as the body of Christ active in the world. Butch grew up wanting to do some good with his life. He doesn't have any power over tsunamis or hurricanes, but he does have power over his choice to work in a place committed to a healing ministry that touches lives in his own city.

Churches face the question of what a healing ministry looks like and come up with answers that fit their situations. It might be a monthly free medical clinic during which Sunday school rooms transform into exam rooms and the fellowship hall is a waiting room. It might be congregations banding together to offer a children's wellness clinic before the start of each school year and give kids shots, screenings, and school supplies. It might be commitment to regular financial and volunteer support at a community clinic that touches the lives of people who would never come through a church door. It might be a parish nurse who makes herself available to people in the congregation for questions in times of wellness and a comforting presence in times of illness.

A congregational health ministry does not require medical professionals in the congregation. When I spent a summer in Zimbabwe during medical school, I encountered the concept of the village health care worker. Usually this is a woman who already has the trust of the community. Perhaps she goes through a simple training process covering basic health care issues, and now she works as the eyes and ears of the professional health care person in that area. She may be the first to identify someone who needs care and make sure it happens.

We've taken this model into the churches of Memphis with a church health promoter ministry. Virtually every church has someone—usually a woman—who has the trust of the congregation on multiple levels. People are already going to her for advice. The Church Health Center offers an eight-week training program on basic topics. We cover community resources people may not be aware of, nutrition, mental and emotional health, common health issues such as hypertension and diabetes, and basic understanding of medications. We look at prenatal, well baby, and women's issues. We stare sexually transmitted disease in the face—yes, in the church. When they finish the training, these people become the eyes and ears of health care in the congregation. Like the women in the African villages, they may be the first to see an unmet health care need and respond to it.

A seventeen-year-old boy fell off a roof while working as a roofer and ended up at our clinic. His injured arm wasn't healing. It turned out he had broken two bones. As I looked at the x-ray and talked with him, my first thought was, *You're seventeen. Why aren't you in school? Why are you working?* I was jumping to conclusions. As we talked, I learned that when his family first came to Memphis, his father died in a traffic accident. Then his mother developed breast cancer. He had three younger siblings at home and was now the primary breadwinner for the family. He did what needed to be done because it was right, and he's a lesson to the rest of us.

Individuals, whether medical professionals or not, can take on a conviction of wellness just the way this young man took on the conviction that it was his job to provide for the family. We can model wellness to family and friends beyond fixing what breaks. We can help others pursue wellness in their own lives because God created them body-and-spirit. That is the healing presence of the gospel, God's kingdom power at work in real lives.

Nancy is a master gardener at the Church Health Center who volunteers considerable time and extensive skill to make the grounds around our center attractive. Her conviction is that even a bed of well-tended flowers or a striking arrangement of bushes offers a picture of healing, and even the poor deserve to come to a beautiful place. Their healing doesn't start when they see the doctor's face. It is all around them when they come to see us. Patients stop and talk to her as she works, and she has her own personal healing presence in direct contact as well as in her fastidious work.

We just have to do it. Most of us spend far too much time trying to match our insides with other people's outsides. We see someone who seems calm and collected and think, *I'm a wreck. How can she be so composed?* That person probably is a wreck, too! You just can't see inside. We're all in this together. People seek a fruitful life characterized by joy and love. Many never find it, often because they remain isolated and do not experience the benefits of community. The most fundamental asset the church can offer to people in need is its existence as a caring community. The body of Christ. God's kingdom presence.

This is not rocket science. It's not a trick question. Living is hard, but no one should have to do it alone. How can you be a healing presence?

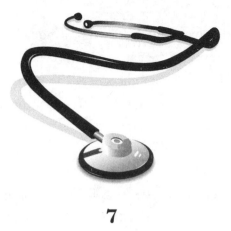

7

Life Is More Than a Heartbeat

Life's too short to take the ugly way home.

I love a parade. I always have. A parade makes me joyous for no particular reason other than watching people celebrate. My favorite, without question, is the Macy's Thanksgiving Day Parade in New York. Growing up in Atlanta, I used to watch it on television every year, without fail. During seminary at Yale, I had a friend who lived in New York. I confessed my love of the Thanksgiving Day Parade, and he reluctantly agreed to take me home with him for Thanksgiving so we could go to the parade.

When the great day came, my friend dawdled around in the morning far longer than I felt necessary, but we finally headed downtown. He decided to stop for an errand; then something else occurred to him, and something else. I, of course, fixated on the clock. Precious parade minutes ticked by, and I could do nothing about it. Finally we arrived at the parade route—just in time to see a dozen men jumping up and down on Bullwinkle's head to deflate the balloon.

Not the morning I had in mind.

But the imagery of this experience is the perfect picture of the way many people live their lives. They constantly pull in a direction *away* from joy. They spurn every suggestion for how they might move *toward* joy. Life for them is about getting the errands done. But avoiding the things that bring joy to you and to others is no way to live. You're just jumping on Bullwinkle's head to get the parade over with.

We are—body-and-spirit—created and loved by God, and in our humanity we experience a spectrum of emotions that is the stuff of life—joy, love, happiness, frustration, anger, despair. The church, the body of Christ, has the opportunity to be the community that cares about all these things and to be a healing presence announcing God's presence in the midst of them. But still we struggle with the meaning of life. Or rather, we struggle to pursue true life—an experience of joy and love that drives us closer to God.

My wife often says, "Life's too short to take the ugly way home." When we get wrapped up in being busy, getting things done, accomplishing something, or just surviving, we miss the beauty of our human experience. We miss life. We fixate on quantity—of years, of possessions, of accomplishments—and we miss the whole parade of joy that is life.

Celebrate you. Celebrate God.

A man came to the Church Health Center's new patient clinic. He used to sell bonds for a living and earned over a hundred thousand dollars a year. Then he got laid off. He spent a year trying to find another job with the same level of income and came up with nothing. In the meantime, his savings dwindled. The stress on his family intensified his wife's bipolar disorder, and the state of his marriage was nothing short of disaster. And in the middle of this, he developed macular degeneration, a serious vision disease. He ended up taking a job as an assistant manager at a fast-food restaurant.

This paid some of the bills, but the job offered no health benefits, so he turned up at our clinic.

"I can't see," he said. "I can't afford medicine. My marriage is a wreck. I have a pile of bills." Then he sat back in his chair, folded his arms across his chest, and stared at me. Dared me. "Can you help me?"

I paused. His troubles were overwhelming. "Yes, we can," I said. "That's what we do."

I could get him to the best eye doctor in Memphis, arrange for a marital counselor, and treat his wife's bipolar disorder. I could offer him the opportunity to use our Wellness facility on a regular basis and benefit from both exercise and community. I could not give him back his high-income job, nor restore his lost sight, but I could help him with things that mattered to the core of his sense of wellness. I could help him see that he could still be happy, still experience joy.

People are always thinking of all the things they should have done, the things they wish they had done. They often think they would do things differently if they could do them again. But when the road lies ahead of you, meandering toward the things you're going to do, it's easy to veer off the path. It's easy to detour to the errands and miss the parade. Very few people have the ability to be fully in the present moment, rather than running through a steady mental inventory of things yet to be done before the day is over.

Sharon, who works in our Wellness facility, has always had a strong faith. On a trip to Israel, she attended a healing service. Everyone seemed to participate in some way. Sharon was not aware of any need she had for healing, but the priest said, "Just come up for the blessing," so she did. Exactly one week later, Sharon discovered she had breast cancer. At the time of the healing service, she had not yet found the lump. In some ways, though, because of the healing service she felt she was healed already. She simply had to go through the process of surgery, chemotherapy, and radiation. Through it all, she had a sense that she was healed.

The experience of illness brought Sharon lessons she might not otherwise have seen. She learned it was okay to let others care for her—drive carpools, cook dinners, and so on. She also learned it was okay to say no. She did not have to do everything, be everything for everybody. In the midst of that illness, Sharon decided, "I'm not going to waste my time doing things that don't have a purpose or bring me joy. Life is full of too many wonderful things to surround myself with negative people." Sharon understood that life is not about being cancer free. Life is about noticing the beauty on the way home, even if it takes you out of your way. Life is about running toward the parade, not detouring for the errands. Life is about finding joy in the parade, not seeing it as a pointless nuisance. Life is about being really *there* in the moment you are in.

Being fully present in the moment includes being fully present to God. Most Christians don't have a real concept of Sabbath these days. They have a concept of the weekend—it's a time to cram in everything we didn't do during the week because we were working. Weekends fill up with chores and catching up around home. Going to church too often becomes one more chore. We miss the opportunity to fully give ourselves over to God, even for one day. We miss the time to remember who we really are—body-and-spirit, created and loved by God.

One of the reasons I think everybody should celebrate their birthday is because it's the one day of the year that people acknowledge your value in just being you, and not because of what you do. The reason to celebrate is just because you were born, just because you *are*. Sabbath is the same kind of experience. We honor the Sabbath because it is God's day, and the point is we get to be with God. We celebrate our connection to God. That's all the day has to be about. If we don't plan for it, however, it will never happen.

Until the last forty years or so, Americans regarded Sunday as a near-mandatory Sabbath. Activity stopped. Blue laws kept stores closed. Mothers made sure their families went to church. Children's sports leagues cleared out of the parks for the day. Now Sunday is a day of more work, only slightly different than the rest of the week. Sunday morning is another slot to cram in a Little League game. We think the world will spin out of control if we sit back and do nothing for a while. The result is a dangerously fatigued nation doing errands on the way to the parade and never seeing the parade.

I've been teaching an adult Sunday school class at St. John's United Methodist Church in Memphis for more than two decades. From time to time, someone asks me why I keep teaching the class, because surely it's one more demand in a packed schedule. But preparing to teach is a time of meditation for me. It gives me an opportunity to ponder things that have nothing to do with the Church Health Center and focus on my own relationship with God. Other people in the class feed me. After twenty-five years, I still look forward to it. If I have to be away on a Sunday, I miss being with the group of people with whom I have an intense connection.

I feel no guilt whatsoever about the fact that virtually every Sunday afternoon, after church, you can find me on the couch with my wife, reading. We do nothing of consequence all afternoon, with our dogs at our feet. Late in the day we might work in the yard, though the point is not to accomplish anything but simply to enjoy the day.

God did not make the human body to go full speed for eighteen hours a day, seven days a week. How many e-mails do you get from friends who send them at two in the morning? We never stop. Religious or not, we need planned rest, a day to turn off the computer and television and turn our brains to the things that bring us joy.

If I miss a Sunday of Sabbath, I pay the price for the whole next week. I am not fully myself again until I have another Sabbath. A regular experience of stepping back nourishes my connection to God and restores wellness to body-and-spirit. This spills into all the aspects of my life. As human beings, we are far more effective and generally fun to be around if we are well rested. We can offer our best to our work and relationships, rather than showing up cranky and aloof and ready to stomp on Bullwinkle's head.

Celebrate the rapids.

Sometimes we have the most profound growing experiences when we least expect them, when they don't fit into carefully laid plans. We may see the beauty of our lives—joy and love—in moments that were never on our list of things to do.

When I was a senior in high school, my mother was diagnosed with ovarian cancer. She had surgery, and the doctors told my father and me that she would probably live another ten years. As a physician now, I don't know why they ever said that. A few months later, she had another crisis and died a few weeks later. During the summer between her surgery and death, she was incredibly sick as the cancer advanced and she coped with the side effects of chemotherapy. Still, I did something that summer I did every year, something I loved doing. My friends and I planned a rafting trip on a river in North Carolina.

And then one day my mother said, "Can I go with you?"

My mother on a rafting trip with my teenage friends? Every young man's dream.

I swallowed hard and said, "Sure." And she went with us.

At the end of the river was one mammoth rapid. Right before we got to it, the guide pulled the raft to the edge of the river so we could scout the rapid and make a plan for going through it. My mother got scared. Safely out of the boat, she thought she would just stay at the side of the river and not go through this last rapid. And then she surprised me again and said, "Why not?" and got back in the raft, and we headed for the last rapid.

I leaned the wrong direction at a critical moment. When I should have leaned forward, I leaned backward, and in the blink of an eye I was out of the raft and in the water. Almost as fast, my mother reached out and grabbed me. She and a friend pulled me back into the raft. Probably I was in the water less than ten seconds. And then we were through the rapid and the trip was over.

This experience has hovered in my life all these years as a powerful metaphor. While my mother clearly was dying, she reached out and pulled me back into the boat. We're not always sure whom we need to depend on to help us stay in the boat. I didn't expect my mother—especially while seriously ill—to raft a river with me, but I was glad she was there. My mother didn't skip the last rapid. She got back in the boat because she loved me, and she was there to reach out one more time to do what mothers do. She gave me what I needed at that moment. We all need to live our lives that way, with a willingness to go down the river in the boat with the people we love. If somebody falls out of the boat, we reach out and pull the person back in.

We need to be more comfortable with being uncertain. We don't always know what the river will do. Uncertainty gives us the opportunity for growth. The human experience always offers more to enrich our lives, more to learn. Too many people grow to a certain point and then they stop. That's who they are for the rest of their lives. I find that sad. People who are not learning more about themselves and more about their faith in the midst of their life experiences do not continue to grow closer to God. We have enormous opportunities to fill our lives with joy, to see the parade— even to march in the parade.

My dear friend Howard was eighty-five years old when he lost his wife. For sixty-five years they were *Howard-and-Margaret.* Then Margaret developed an unusual form of lung cancer and died in a fairly short period of time. By then, Howard was in his mideighties. They shared a profound, rich love that is a burning image in my life. Now he had to figure out how to be just *Howard.* It was a little scary, but even at eighty-five Howard thought, *God is giving me a chance to figure out who Howard is. How can I build off my love for Margaret and make myself a better person?* He stayed in the parade.

Don't hide the Cross.

Bill Muehl was a professor of preaching at Yale Divinity School for twenty years. I once heard him tell the story of a Christmas pageant at church when his children were young. His six-year-old son was cast as a shepherd. The play included two Virgin Marys, three Josephs, five wise men, a cluster of little girl angels, and a pack of little boy shepherds.

At the last rehearsal, everything went smoothly and all the kids knew what to do. At the performance, the two Virgin Marys took their places and were as beautiful as could be. The three Josephs were stoic and stood where they were supposed to stand. The five wise men approached regally. The angels were as radiant as angels ever have been and took their places exactly where they were supposed to in the tableau. Then came the shepherds, and chaos broke out. The shepherds treated the angels in ways no one ever treated angels before. Little girls were being tossed around the stage. My professor recognized the six-year-old voice that rose above it all. "All these stupid angels have hidden my cross."

It turned out that everyone on the stage had a cross-mark to stand on. The final rehearsal was not a dress rehearsal, so it was easy to see the marks. During the performance, however, the billowy gowns the angels were wearing hid the shepherds' marks. Dresses hid the crosses and the shepherds couldn't find where they were supposed to stand.

How unbelievably true of the tableau of our lives. We may have everything in its place and it's a magnificent picture, but somehow we manage to hide the Cross. Our lives do not reflect what Jesus' death and resurrection actually mean to us. We don't want to see the brutality of the cross, so we hide it with the satiny aspects of our lives. We're not willing to gaze into the face of what sickness, suffering, and death can mean to us and see that even they can bring beauty to our lives.

Robert worked as a yardman for a doctor who volunteered for the Church Health Center. His boss noticed he was losing weight and lacked his usual energy. Robert also had a slight cough and some diarrhea. When I did a physical exam, I felt large lymph nodes in his neck and groin. This was in 1988. The AIDS epidemic was in full swing, and with no drugs yet available to treat it, AIDS was a death sentence.

When I told Robert he had AIDS, he did not blink an eye. He thanked me. Over the next year, I saw Robert every two months. He continued to lose weight and the lymph nodes grew larger. Even though he lost energy, he showed up for work. What never changed was his attitude toward life. He was joyous about the people in his life. In fact, he was concerned that I was working too hard.

After seeing Robert like this on several occasions, I wondered if he understood the dire circumstances of his diagnosis. His life was ending, and the last few months would be agonizing. So one day as he cheerfully told me about the good things in his life, I stopped him. I looked him in the eye and said, "Robert, do you understand that you have AIDS and there is no cure for this illness?" Robert took me by the hand and said, "Yes, Doc, I understand what is wrong with me. I also know that God loves me."

I realized Robert understood far more about life and living than

I did. As a physician and a Methodist minister, at that point in time I saw health primarily as the absence of disease, and I did not fully understand the need for joy, love, and the assurance of God's presence in order to be fully alive. Although Robert died six months later, he taught me a great deal about what a healthy life entails. His desire to work hard, do a good job, love his friends, and live in constant devotion to God led him to be happy and know joy even while dying of AIDS.

I no longer see health as the mere absence of disease. Health is built around community and grounded in the spiritual life that embraces the physical bodies God gives us. Instead of the absence of disease, I see health as the presence of those elements that lead us to joy and love and drive us closer to God. Living longer is not the goal for a healthy life. Rather, loving fully, with all our capacity, will define a well-lived life.

Life is more than keeping your heart beating and your lungs breathing. We get bound up in the technological explanations of life—heartbeat, brain waves, respiration. We get bound up in the demands and expectations of life, whether that means astounding accomplishment or simply making it through the day. But those things do not tell you whether you are well and healthy.

Don't skip the rapids. The rapids are invitations to joy and love and the presence of God. Life's too short to take the ugly way home.

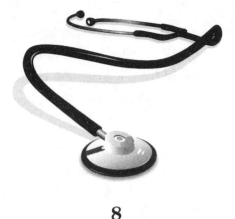

8

Who's the Real Enemy?

You're going to die. (But it won't be today.)

"What do you think is going to happen?" Frank asked me on the telephone.

Frank's wife, Gloria, was in a coma and on a ventilator for forty days following an accident. Her kidneys had failed. Nothing about her medical condition gave reason to hope for recovery.

"If she has a living will," I said, "we need to get it. If she didn't want her life excessively extended by artificial means, we need to honor her wishes."

"But what constitutes 'excessive'?" Frank countered.

"This does, Frank," I answered softly. "Forty days on a ventilator. That's excessive."

His voice cracked over the phone line, as though the truth was hitting him for the first time. "She's going to die, isn't she?"

I closed my eyes before I answered. "I think that's what will happen, Frank. I'm so sorry."

We hung up, and I felt terrible. Had I been too direct? Should I have held out some hope? The possibility of any recovery was remote beyond reason. Yet I hated to have to tell Frank.

As much as we don't understand about life, we instinctively value it and cling to it. When death threatens loved ones, we don't want to let go. Death is the enemy, and we will fight to the end.

But *is* death the enemy? When we embrace the beauty of our body-and-spirit humanity, in all its complexities, perhaps we can also embrace the complex thought that death is not the enemy.

Death is part of life.

I used to say to patients something like, "You're going to die, but it won't be today." After all, everyone is going to die. One day a patient called my nurse, sobbing over the news I had given her the day before that she was dying. I had to get on the phone then and try to explain that it was a joke, a light remark. The patient did not see the humor, to say the least, and I stopped saying that to patients. Clearly the thought of dying strikes fear in the hearts of many people.

Mrs. Garcia didn't speak English, so her daughter did the talking when they came to see me. Mrs. Garcia had undergone surgery in Mexico about six months earlier, and her daughter arranged for her to come into the United States legally in order to seek further medical care. "They say she has cancer," her daughter explained. "She needs a liver transplant, but they won't give it to her."

My mind began to spin. If what she said was true, how could I use our resources for someone who was already being treated in another country and apparently had an advanced disease? But this woman traveled thousands of miles in search of hope. I did a physical exam, which confirmed that her liver disease was severe, and chose my words carefully as I spoke to Mrs. Garcia's daughter.

"I do not think I am going to be able to do anything that doctors in Mexico cannot do. Also, I'm worried that if she stays here and has to be in the hospital, she might receive a very large bill." I tried to speak kindly, but the daughter began to cry.

"If she goes back to Mexico," she said, "they will just let her die because she is old."

We discussed medications and I did some blood work. Things did not add up. There was no sign of cancer. Instead, she had cirrhosis of the liver, probably from hepatitis. Yet she still needed a transplant.

"Your mother has a very serious disease," I told the daughter. "A transplant might help if she were younger, but she is sixty-three and a citizen of Mexico. I don't believe she could receive a liver transplant in this country."

The daughter replied, "They said it would take a long time if she stayed in Mexico." Tears welled in her eyes.

I was stunned. Mrs. Garcia was already on a transplant list. Her doctors were doing everything I would do. But her daughter was fighting her mother's death with every remote possibility she could muster.

Our love affair with technology pushes us to fend off death at all costs. We fight death with technology, even extreme technology. In reality, though, people want to die with dignity, surrounded by their family and friends who care for them. "Do everything you can" is not necessarily the right thing to do. However, most likely we will keep doing it until we have the right conversations about the meaning of life, rather than the wrong conversations about the best technology. Mrs. Garcia and her daughter needed to have the right conversation. Christians must be willing to engage in the right conversation with their own families as well as the culture around them. An understanding of real life allows us to let go of hating death as the enemy.

Death does not win.

One of the most powerful passages in the New Testament on the theme of death is in 2 Corinthians. Paul opens this letter with a moving relational picture of God as "the Father of compassion and the God of all comfort." In our sufferings, God comforts us. Paul then defends his own ministry, which grew out of his deeply personal experience of God's mercy, and the utterly firm hope that is within us because believers are connected to God. Paul reminds his readers in Corinth, and us through the Word of God, that we are being transformed into Christ's likeness with ever-increasing glory. God's own creative light shines in our hearts. And then comes the glorious passage from chapter 4 that we often read at funerals as an assurance of eternal life after death. We also should embrace it in life as an assurance of God's presence in the here and now.

> But we have this treasure in jars of clay to show that this all-surpassing power is from God and not from us. We are hard pressed on every side, but not crushed; perplexed, but not in despair; persecuted, but not abandoned; struck down, but not destroyed. We always carry around in our body the death of Jesus, so that the life of Jesus may also be revealed in our body. . . . With that same spirit of faith we also believe and therefore speak, because we know that the one who raised the Lord Jesus from the dead will also raise us with Jesus. (2 Corinthians 4:7–14)

Ordinary clay jars of the first century sometimes carried treasure. Paul's imagery is concrete, not some vague philosophy. Our body-and-spirit existence carries the treasure of the light of God. We don't receive this treasure when we die; we live with it. Our bodily lives reveal Jesus' life, and Jesus' life was an announcement of the kingdom of God. He brought a radical understanding of health and wholeness that comes from being connected to God. No matter what happens in our body-and-spirit humanity, God does not abandon us. Our troubles, our disappointments, the failures of our physical bodies—all point to God at work in us. We live in that reality, even now.

And in the end, the kingdom of God triumphs. God raised Jesus from the dead, and God will raise us. Death will not have the final victory. God will, and we will share in it. "The trumpet will sound," Paul says, and "the dead will be raised" (1 Corinthians 15:52). Death already has been swallowed up in victory. "Where, O death, is your victory?" Paul asks. "Where, O death, is your sting?" (1 Corinthians 15:55).

Do we grieve? Absolutely. Do we feel loss? Keenly. Do we lose the battle for meaning because death is part of the human body-and-spirit experience? Resoundingly, no. Who better than Christians to lead the conversation about the meaning of life and the place of death in our human experience?

In the United States, we don't have sufficient conversation on these questions because we are too busy fighting death with technology. More than a quarter of Medicare's budget is spent during the last six months of people's lives. Many people spend up to 80 percent of their lifetime medical expenses in the last six months of life. We sit idly by while people suffer needlessly in the hope of living for brief periods of time that are often spent in loud, aseptic intensive care units away from their loved ones.

A cultural moral conversation doesn't happen in a year or in a presidential term or perhaps even in a generation. It likely won't happen at all if the church does not step forward to lead it. In the meantime, though, families can have this conversation. Rather than keep people alive in a coma and on a ventilator for forty days, rather than chase technology and knowledge across international borders, let's start talking about valuing life enough to embrace even death as a vehicle of God's grace in our lives. I am not speaking about isolated instances of euthanasia or withholding care, as if a human agent should decide if a person lives or dies. I'm looking at the much bigger principle of living and dying with dignity and believing that God is with us even in death. As Christians we say we believe that, yet we don't always make choices consistent with that belief. Let's start talking about it. Death is not the enemy. Jesus conquered death.

I remember a day when I saw two relatively recent widows on the same day in the clinic. Nancy's husband had died eight months earlier from cancer after it manifested in several parts of his body and doctors treated it each time.

"They never told us he was terminal," Nancy said to me. "They never put him in the hospital. The doctor said it was better for him to stay home than be in the hospital, so we had to watch him die."

"We had to watch him die." Would Nancy rather have left her husband to die alone in the hospital? I'm not sure.

The very next patient that day was Rachel, whose husband had died about a year and a half earlier.

"I know it's been hard for you," I said as I patted her leg.

"It would have been a lot worse," she said, "except for the comfort my Master gave me. I heard the Lord say to me, 'Give him back. I loaned him to you for forty-seven years, and now he's coming home to me.' "

I had no doubt Rachel felt her husband was with God, and that was a great comfort. She responded with joy while Nancy felt overwhelming despair.

God remains in control.

Years ago I had a partner at the Church Health Center, Dr. Febe Wallace. She had a little boy named Scott, whom we all watched grow to the age of three. While Febe and her family were away for a ski vacation in Utah, Scott got sick, rapidly and severely. Febe and Tom found a local pediatrician and insisted on checking Scott's white blood count, which turned out to be very high. In a horrifying sequence of events, they realized that Scott had leukemia. They came right home to Memphis to have Scott treated at St. Jude Children's Research Hospital. It wasn't long before they knew Scott had a form of leukemia that is much more challenging to treat successfully than the more common form. They began chemotherapy, and Scott's numbers improved. Then suddenly this precious little boy had a massive stroke.

All this happened in a matter of days, and Febe and Tom were faced with a difficult decision. Scott was on a ventilator with his eyes closed. Febe stroked his head while she spoke calmly and told me what was going on. "He has a huge bleed, and even if he survives this, he will be left with a major deficit. Then we still have to treat him for the leukemia. We have a window of opportunity to let him go, and we think we need to take it."

Febe and Tom made the brave decision not to put their hope in technology but in God. Febe did not want Scott to suffer a single minute longer than necessary because she was holding out hope for improvement that was extremely unlikely. She put his welfare and comfort ahead of her need to grasp at the odds. The family gathered, and Febe held her son as the doctor removed the breathing tube and turned off the ventilator. It took only a few minutes for Scott to take his last breath. It was one of the most heart-wrenching moments of my life.

"I know he is in a better place," Febe said to me. "I can only trust that God knows better than we do." She held on to her conviction that God remained in control, and Scott's death was not meaningless, even though she could not express its purpose at that moment. Certainly his short life was full of purpose and joy and love.

Do we believe God is present in all aspects of our body-and-spirit humanity? I don't want to hear platitude answers any more than the next person. However, our view of death is one place where it gets increasingly harder to view religion and science as separate tracks, both true, that never intersect. At what point will we understand that technology does not give meaning to life? God does. If we believe that while living, we must believe it while dying.

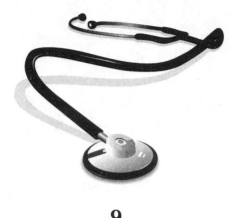

9

The Whole You Can Find Peace

Wellness is what happens when you drink of the well.

At first I thought I was looking at the wrong chart. The patient in front of me looked like she was in her forties, but the chart said she was sixty-six. Just to be sure, I asked her age.

"I'm sixty-six," she said, "but my children keep me looking young." She giggled like a schoolgirl.

I was curious now. "How many children do you have?"

"Sixteen. Eleven girls and five boys."

"Oh my," I said. "I'd like to meet their father."

"Well, I had eight by my first husband and eight by my second."

"I guess you've spent most of your life taking care of children."

"Yes, sir," she said, nodding. "That, and working in the fields."

"So you worked on a farm?"

"I picked cotton most of my life, until the boss bought a cotton-picking machine. That knocked me out."

"It sounds to me like you've had a pretty hard life."

"No, sir," Mary replied immediately. "I've had a good life. God has been good to me."

I went home that day hoping some of Mary's view of life had rubbed off on me.

Evelyn lost both her legs and now struggled for her life. In the course of a few days, she seemed to face one crisis after another. She was in a coma, and we weren't sure what was going to happen. Her kidneys weren't working, and her bowel was troublesome. A week or so later, she seemed to stabilize, and eventually she recovered enough to go home after four weeks in the hospital. Medically her case remained complicated, though.

A month or so later I saw her at the clinic—looking very good. She laughed as she rolled by me in her wheelchair. Her daughter's marriage was collapsing, and her daughter and granddaughter had moved in with Evelyn and her husband. Evelyn now spent much of her time taking care of the baby.

"Maybe that's why God saved me," she said, "because I'm needed to help raise this baby. You know I nearly died, but I'm almost a walking miracle." She paused and looked down at her stumps. "Well, if I could walk, I'd be a walking miracle!"

After everything she went through, Evelyn found forward-looking purpose. Physically, her own life was not easy by any stretch of the imagination, and now she faced added family stress. But she responded by finding purpose, not despair. From her perspective, her life overflowed with joy and love and purpose—the real stuff of life.

Health is not the absence of disease.

Being disease free does not make you healthy. In fact, disease has little to do with whether a person is well. Instead, wellness has to do with whether the person can see God's presence in a way that draws the person forward into the glory of the kingdom of God. Wellness embraces the joy of living then acts in a way that allows for thriving in happiness, love, and closeness to God. Wellness is what happens when you drink of the well.

Jesus went out of his way to meet a Samaritan woman at a well that served a small village. He dispatched his disciples on a quest for food and cleared the scene for a private conversation. Jesus knew this woman was far from perfect. In fact, her life was in the shocking and scandalous category. So much was wrong with it. Five former husbands, a live-in lover: Shame took her to the well at the hottest part of the day so she wouldn't have to face nosy neighbors. A good Jewish man like Jesus ought to have known better than to talk to any Samaritan woman, and especially this one. But Jesus wasn't looking for a reason for judgment; he was offering a reason for joy. Jesus offered himself as "living water" to this woman—"a spring of water welling up to eternal life" (John 4:11, 14).

Notice that Jesus did not present himself as a quiet, placid stream that might lull you into an afternoon snooze. Neither is he still water that turns brackish over time. He is a vigorous, robust, gushing fountain that would carry the woman to God. Abundant life—that's what Jesus was talking about. It's the whole reason he came to share our body-and-spirit humanity. Jesus was willing to forgive the woman for everything she had ever done if she was willing now to look for a life that embraced the goodness and richness of the path he set before her.

In an impromptu teaching time on a mountainside with a crowd listening in, Jesus said essentially, "Don't worry about your life. Watch the birds. Stop to smell the roses. Quit wasting your energy fretting about the details of your day-to-day existence, and pay attention to what God is doing."

Above all else, this is what we need. I see a lot of patients who live from paycheck to paycheck, but rather than worrying through each day, they strive to live each day. Most of what we worry about is beyond our control. Endless worrying about the stock market doesn't change the stock market. And most of what we worry about never happens anyway. I don't mean to sound like a Pollyanna, but the message that God is present in the midst of the troubles of this world can be a healing balm. "See how the lilies of the field grow," Jesus said. Whether you live in the asphalt jungle of New York or the desert of North Africa, the lilies of the field are the things that bring hope into your life and touch on beauty. They are the things that lift your eyes from your immediate challenges to a bigger picture of God's work in the world. They are the things that stir up your faith. Those things exist no matter where you are. You can find God's healing presence in order to live joyfully today. You can be broken and still be healthy.

We cannot separate faith from the rest of us.

My friend Gary Gunderson, author of *Leading Causes of Life*, has been exploring the connections between faith and health for about as long as I have. In this pursuit, he visited the southern African country of Lesotho. Gary and his team developed a questionnaire to guide their research, but they ran into immediate trouble when they discovered that the Sesotho language of the people they were studying did not separate the concept of faith from health. Questions that treated faith and health as separate were meaningless to the people who were supposed to answer them.

Whether Sesotho speakers use the word we translate *health* or the word for *faith*, the other is always in the back of the mind. They do not speak of one without also meaning the other. They do, however, have a word that reflects their concept of the wholeness of life. *Bophelo* is an intricate network of relationships with family and community, with land and creation, with the seen and the unseen. This totality of relationships is the source of bophelo. While we in the West have thought of health as a piece of us that we can separate out from the rest of our lives, the people of Lesotho have known all along that we experience life as a whole. We use the

English word *alive* largely to mean a biological state in contrast to death, but *bophelo*—the root means "alive"—refers to being in a state of wellness in all the dimensions of life. The most common greeting among the Sesotho people—the equivalent of our "How are you?"—uses the root of *bophelo*. It means "How are you living?" or "How alive are you?" It speaks to the person as a whole, not to a physical piece or some other piece that could somehow be broken off from the whole. If we had an English word that meant "life-ness" or "living-ness," that would be bophelo.

I see patients every day who do not have a diagnosis I can label, but in my gut I know they are not healthy. They are missing joy or happiness or even simple kindness from their lives. One woman was so certain she was sick that every time I reassured her that her symptoms were not a sign of serious illness, she came up with yet another pain she was just sure indicated a terrible disease. When I emphatically told her we could help her best through Church Health Center Wellness, a facility that helps people improve wellness in all the aspects of their lives, she barked at me, "You'd rather see me be happy exercising than treat me for my misery."

Her statement was right on target. Her misery was linked fundamentally to her lack of wellness in spirit. She was unhealthy, but it was not simply a matter of something gone wrong in the body. Treating the body only was not going to make her healthy. Her best chance at feeling less miserable physically was learning to see herself as *body-and-spirit*, rather than trying to treat one part of her without seeing the whole of her life and being. Some simple exercise at our Wellness facility could have been the first step toward understanding why she felt miserable.

The biblical concept of *shalom* is a powerful argument that God cares about the well-being of people. This word appears in the Old Testament more than 250 times and overwhelmingly points to well-being that comes from God in the widest sense of the word.

Shalom describes not only a spiritual connection to God, but a life connection—bodily health, contentedness, social relationships. Everything that God gives us in all aspects of our lives comes under the umbrella of shalom. Completeness, wholeness, fullness—these are all at the heart of shalom. God gave Moses a blessing to pass on to the people that culminates in shalom:

> The LORD bless you and keep you;
>> the LORD make his face shine upon you and be
>> gracious to you;
>> the LORD turn his face toward you and give you peace.
> (Numbers 6:24–26)

Shalom. God's peace. Many churches observe the ancient Christian practice of "sharing the peace." One person says, "The peace of the Lord be with you," and the response comes, "And also with you." When we say this, we are not simply saying, "Good morning! Isn't it a lovely day!" The words are profound blessing. "May your life be full of God! May you live in the joy of being connected to God!" *Sharing* the peace means we seek to live in God's wholeness together, as a faith community.

The prophet Isaiah spoke of the Messiah to come as the Prince of Peace, the embodiment of shalom (Isaiah 9:6). Jesus, the fulfillment of the prophecy, brought the kingdom of God to the here and now and showed us a transformed reality. When Jesus healed, he brought faith and health together. Healing of body-and-spirit pointed to God's active presence in the world. Early Christians formed a community to be God's active healing presence in the world—the body of Christ—and to run after God's healing priorities in the world together.

I am convinced that true health always occurs through a community experience. When people live out their faith together, the health of everyone who shares the experience is enhanced. In the Judeo-Christian tradition, health is a holistic concept that reflects a person's relationship to God. Churches, for instance, help people experience life through the joy of knowing God. Working together in the world in order to experience God's love makes us healthy. This vision of health can be reality even when someone has a disease of the body.

Bring faith into your story of wellness.

A woman who suffered for twelve years with a continuous illness followed Jesus. She went to the doctors. Lots of them. The Talmud, an ancient Jewish teaching text, contains medicines and treatments prescribed for the kind of illness the woman had, and no doubt she tried them all in twelve years. But she got worse, not better. Now she was ready to bring faith into the story. This woman heard about Jesus, but she didn't want to be too much trouble. She thought, "If I just touch his clothes, I will be healed" (Mark 5:28). Her faith gave her hope when nothing else did. When she managed to graze Jesus' clothing as he walked by, she "felt in her body that she was freed from her suffering" (5:29).

Despite the woman's subtle action of touching the cloak of a man in motion, Jesus knew something happened, and he was determined to find out who touched him. The woman was petrified, but she told the truth. Jesus said, "Daughter, your faith has healed you. Go in peace and be freed from your suffering" (5:34).

Faith, healing, peace, freedom from suffering—all in one brief encounter. Jesus did not separate faith from health. Jesus did not disassemble the whole person God created and leave the parts lying around in separate piles. Jesus interacted with the whole person. He blessed the woman with shalom, the peace of God.

God wants this kind of wholeness and wellness for you. God created you, body-and-spirit. Jesus came and shared our existence so you could have a full, meaningful life. God is present in the world through the body of Christ, and you don't have to be alone. Even in great suffering—even in death—God is there. The whole you can experience peace that brings healing to your life, not just what might be broken in your body at the moment.

Like the woman who suffered for twelve years, perhaps you are ready to reach out for a new level of well-being in your life, a well-being that springs out of being connected to God.

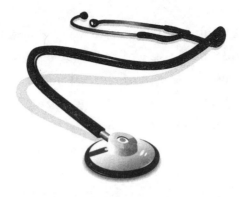

10

Health Care Change Starts with You

The quality of our intervention programs matches the quality of technology a hundred years ago.

Mamie had not been to the clinic in seven or eight years, so I began by asking her, "Have you been doing okay or have you been going to another doctor?"

She nonchalantly replied, "Oh, I've been doing pretty good. The WD40 has kept my knees oiled, but it doesn't seem to work anymore."

I laughed, thinking it was a joke, then realized Mamie wasn't the sort of person who makes jokes. She really was using a mechanical lubricant on her knees. And frankly, that's not the strangest story I've heard over the years.

Many people do want to help themselves, but finding the right starting point isn't always easy. We sometimes chase the wrong information because we haven't stopped to ask the right questions.

If God wants wholeness for us as whole beings, what gets in the way of experiencing it? What can I do to remove the obstacles in my own experience?

If a business model of health care does not make people healthier, what would? What can I do to make myself healthier?

What keeps us from making the shifts that would truly reform health care? What shifts do I need to make in my own life?

How do we move from what health care is to what it should be? What kind of health do I want for myself?

What can we do to close the gaps?

Change starts with individuals, not with legislation. Change in your health care starts with you. Health care we can live with starts with growing a new culture that features dignity, community, giving, and prevention.

Dignity matters to health.

An older patient came in with high blood pressure and diabetes, but we got them under control. Everything seemed to be going well. Then he just didn't come back for follow-up visits. When he finally returned, I asked, "Why didn't you come in?" He didn't have the money, plain and simple. On our sliding scale we only asked him to pay ten or fifteen dollars, but he didn't have even that small amount. But he knew he needed to come in, and finally he came up with a solution to his problem.

I watched as he put his hand in a pocket and pulled out a silver dollar. "My mother died since the last time I was here," he explained. "Just before she died she gave me a silver dollar to remember her by for the rest of my life." He pulled out another silver dollar. "My mother gave this one to my brother, and now he's gone, too. He asked me to keep his silver dollar before he died. I can't let you have my brother's silver dollar, but I'll let you have mine."

He held the first silver dollar out toward me, asking me to take it. It was not payment, but it was a guarantee that he would pay the bill. He would never think of leaving his mother's silver dollar with us permanently.

Dignity matters to health.

We need a model for health care that respects the dignity of each person. We need to stop and consider whether we are treating each other with dignity in all our relationships. If I am body-and-spirit, created and loved by God, so are you. We don't earn human dignity—it is a gift from God—and respecting dignity is a gift we can give each other.

Community matters to health.

One of the doctors on our staff at the Church Health Center had a patient who was a little sister of a girl being treated at St. Jude Children's Research Hospital. We often see families connected to St. Jude. One child in the family is a patient there, often for extended periods of time, but the rest of the family must find their health care somewhere else. This family, from Colombia, expected to be in Memphis for several years because of the protocol for treating the older daughter's illness. However, medical visas don't come with work permits. Ricardo asked if he could volunteer for us. He wanted to plug in somewhere and not let his skills sit idle. He wanted to contribute. It turned out he was an amazingly talented computer programmer, something we could really use. It wasn't long before Ricardo was volunteering for us on a full-time basis. His wife was a jack-of-all-trades, and she began to translate for me when I treated Spanish-speaking patients in addition to doing whatever needed to be done around the Church Health Center. Their daughter was seriously ill and they were in a new, strange country. They might easily have withdrawn to focus on their own suffering. Instead, they plunged into a life that would bring wellness to the whole family. Their commitment to the community culture of the Church Health Center was through the roof.

Community matters to health.

We need a model for health care that encourages people to

belong. Whole-life wellness rapidly climbs the chart when people contribute to a community and expand their own social network. We see it all the time in our own Wellness facility. People come together and encourage one another in exercise, nutrition, support groups, and prayer.

And health improves.

Giving matters to health.

A retired United Methodist minister started attending St. John's United Methodist Church, where I am an associate pastor. After the worship service one day, he asked me, "Would you like some of Winnie's babies?" I discovered that Winnie, his wife, often knitted four-inch dolls for her children and grandchildren, and now she wanted to knit babies to give to other children. The kids at the Church Health Center loved them. One day, though, a mother gently asked, "Do you have any that might have a black face?" Winnie had made a pile of tan-faced dolls. She was chagrined that it never crossed her mind to make other colors, but she jumped right in. She made babies in every skin hue you could imagine.

Giving matters to health.

Winnie could have thought she had nothing to offer the Church Health Center because she was not a medical professional, nor in a position to make an enormous financial contribution. But she realized she could give something we never would have known to ask for, and she brought joy to the children who received her gifts.

Prevention matters to health.

When I was in Zimbabwe during medical school, I met the inventor of the VIP, the Ventilated Individual Privy. That simple invention saved as many lives as any medication for malaria or AIDS. A missionary doctor realized that pills were not particularly effective for many conditions because people would get the same water-borne diseases over and over again. Schistosomiasis, for instance, results from standing in water infested with parasites that bore through the feet and invade the bloodstream. The disease affects the liver and is an enormous killer in many parts of the world. The doctor invented a contraption that was both a toilet and a shower. In the morning, the woman of the house would go to the river and bring water back. The water went on the roof of the VIP. During the day, the sun heated the water. When the husband came home in the evening, he could take a hot shower, and the water would run off and filter through the toilet. Heating the water killed the parasites, bathing in the river was unnecessary, and the VIP trapped flies and other insects that spread diseases found in human waste.

This invention came out of the doctor's conversations with the community about what they needed. They themselves recognized that they did not need pills to treat disease, but rather they needed a way to prevent the disease from spreading in the first place.

Prevention matters to health.

Let's ask what make things go *right*, rather than what makes things go *wrong*. Most of prevention has to do with choices that individuals can make for themselves, but people are more likely to make the choices with the help of other people. We know a few things about the physical benefits that come from good nutrition, an active lifestyle, nurturing relationships, and a balanced life. Prevention is not a new word. But research into the benefits of prevention behaviors is in its infancy. The quality of our intervention programs matches the quality of technology a hundred years ago. A century ago we were at the bottom of the technology chart. We are still at the bottom of the prevention chart. The best is still ahead of us if we would focus on it, both in research and in personal action.

A culture of dignity, community, giving, and prevention could revolutionize health care. Those things don't happen by government action. They result from individual choice. Health care change starts with me. It starts with you. We carry each other toward the wellness God created us for.

Start by connecting to God.

Four men, whose names we don't know, took health care into their own hands. A fifth man was paralyzed, and the foursome believed Jesus could do something about it. Jesus was speaking inside a house, but the crowd was so thick the four friends couldn't get anywhere near Jesus. They didn't say, "It can't be done," or "The task requires more resources," or "Why isn't somebody doing something about this?" They banded together, a community of five, and determined to get the job done. Their friend deserved the dignity of seeing Jesus and not being left on the sidelines because of his physical condition. They could not heal his legs themselves, but they had faith that his legs could be healed, and they could contribute by carrying him to Jesus.

So the four men bypassed the crowds, made a hole in the roof, and lowered their ailing friend down to the floor in front of Jesus. The gospel writers tell us Jesus saw their faith. Their drastic method would suggest they had plenty of faith and did not want to miss this opportunity. They expected something from this encounter with Jesus, and Jesus sized up the need pretty fast. "Your sins are forgiven," he said. The religious leaders did not like what they heard, but Jesus did the whole job. First Jesus connected the paralyzed man with God, and then he attended to the physical issue of a body that was not working right. The healed man was an announcement that God was there.

We don't know if the paralyzed man asked his friends for this assistance, but in Acts we read a story of a man who did ask Jesus' followers for help. Unable to walk, this man also was carried, but rather than being carried toward wellness, he was carried to his begging station at the entrance to the temple. When Peter and John arrived, the man begged for money.

Peter and John didn't have any money and said so. I suspect they also knew a few coins were not the man's deepest need for wellness. Peter said he would give what he did have—and he healed the man in the name of Jesus Christ. Feet and ankles that previously could not support any weight now went on a jumping spree—and a praising spree. Not only did the man's body work properly now, but he was connected to God through the experience.

Our lives are healthy when we are linked to a source of meaning—God—and when we experience relationships that sustain us, nurture us, and point us to God over and over again. If you are not convinced of this, you cannot take your health care into your own hands. If you do believe it, though, you have taken the first step toward health care change you can live with.

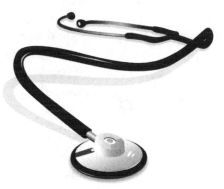

11

Don't Believe
Everything You Hear

If you read it on the Internet, why did you come to see me?

People build careers out of being experts—or at least presenting themselves as experts. They know what you don't know about selling your house or restoring your great-grandmother's clock. They grasp what befuddles you about how your computer talks to itself or how a child learns to read. Navigating the stock market, growing juicier tomatoes, ridding your yard of pesky weeds, getting the stain out of your bathtub, landing an incredible deal on a cruise, building the career of your dreams—pick a topic, and somebody is ready to tell you what you don't know.

Information is everywhere. Have a question? Jump on the Internet and find the answer. As a physician, I hear "I read it on the Internet" all the time. And I think, *If you read it on the Internet, why did you come to see me?* We keep trying to reduce any topic to five easy steps anyone can understand. In addition to words, images are everywhere, and we store their messages in our brains and hearts whether or not anyone says a word. Unfortunately, this all leads to a lot of incomplete or inaccurate—or downright dangerous— information for health care.

What is the real message?

The culture is full of messages that run counter to a true understanding of wellness. Choosing to take your health care into your own hands begins with understanding you are created for a relationship with God. If this is your starting point for recognizing wellness in your own life, you'll begin to distinguish the messages in the culture that work *against* wellness even though buzz words try to convince you they are good for your health.

Here are a few messages that remind us not to believe everything we hear.

Join a gym and get fit! Joining a gym only helps if you go and use the equipment, of course. The membership card doesn't have any special power to do anything but take money out of your bank account every month. But even if you go, a number of things get in the way of success. If you're overweight and out of shape, is seeing yourself from every angle in wall-size mirrors next to some svelte creature in spandex supposed to encourage you to come back tomorrow and subject yourself to that again? Suppose you sit down at a weight machine and discover that the last person who used it was lifting 180 pounds. Perhaps you glance around to make sure no one sees you move the setting down to a basic ten pounds—or you just avoid the weights altogether. Or you get on a treadmill and the electronic display reveals that the previous user ran what seems to you like an infinite distance in an infinitesimal amount of time. Shame is not a great motivator for healthy choices. At our Church Health Center Wellness facility, we don't have mirrors on the wall, our dress code is modest, and our equipment doesn't let anyone see what you are lifting or not lifting.

If you look like this, you'll be happy. Let's face it. The people in those gym ads look like they're taking happy pills and can mysteriously survive for years without eating. The same is true of the sassy commercials and magazine ads full of young, vibrant, athletic models. "Don't I look great?" the faces say. "If you looked as great as I do, you'd be happy, too. Too bad you have the wrong body shape to be happy."

This way of eating will solve all your problems.

Never eat carbohydrates. Stick to protein.

Don't eat any protein, unless it comes from a plant.

Eat carbohydrates, but you have to eat the right ones.

Sugar is the enemy.

Eat no fat whatsoever under any circumstances.

Eat as much as you want—from this list of foods. (If you vary from the list, you fail.)

These scientifically proven foods burn calories without exercise! Just send us $49.99 (plus shipping and handling) for your starter kit.

Nutrition and a healthy weight undoubtedly are important to overall wellness, but we take God's gift of nourishing food and turn it into some kind of contest for how much we can deprive ourselves in the name of being healthy. Eating for wellness should not leave you thinking about food every second of the day—either wishing you could eat something or regretting that you did. We treat food more like a hill to be conquered than an important part of our wellness.

Get thin in just minutes a day! Ten minutes a day gives you the body you've always dreamed of! (And of course once you have this great new body, everything else in your life will fall into place.)

Probably not.

No one piece of machinery, or one food, or one hard-fought

habit is a magic formula for overall wellness. Health is not about shortcuts. Health is about understanding the wholeness God wants for you over a lifetime.

You can do it all. The subtext here is that being busy means you are important. Being independent means you are strong. Accomplishing a lot means you are more valuable than the person who doesn't.

Many people face life circumstances that require them to bear enormous burdens, and I don't make light of that. These people come through our clinic all the time. But they are not happy and well simply because they carry the load. When I point people to our Wellness facility, it's as much for the community as it is for the exercise.

If you're overwhelmed, it's healthy to choose to be less busy.

It's healthy to welcome others into your life to help carry the load.

Heaven does not have an elite subdivision for overachievers who won't accept help.

Technology makes your life easier. What would really happen to your life if you never get an iPad or whatever is coming next? A phone can just be a phone, and it doesn't have to be turned on all the time. A computer can be a tool, not an appendage.

Technology that is supposed to make our lives easier and more enjoyable too often turns into demands. Computers are clearly part of the world we live in, but everything about them hasn't been good. They may make it easier to get the job done, but we lose face-to-face connections. A matter-of-fact e-mail message can cause harm because the personal element is missing. We lose the smile, the pat on the back, the moments that allow us to say, "And how are your kids doing?" Working more because you can work from wherever you are doesn't prove anything. Social networking doesn't replace relationships. Life and health do not happen 140 characters at a time. If technology is isolating you from people and activities that bring you joy, then it's time to take another look at its place in your life.

Faster is better. Often the point of using technology is to do things faster. Why? So we can do more? Why do we need to do more?

The fastest high-speed Internet service.

The fastest car.

The fastest computer.

The fastest route.

The fastest food.

We live our lives at increasingly faster speeds, and it does not make us healthy. Faster is not always better.

You are the expert at taking care of yourself.

This is not an exhaustive list of cultural messages that get in the way of health. No doubt you can add to the list. But any one of these messages can take a chink out of the picture of wholeness that is the core of being healthy. Put several of them together—as most people do every day—and they become disempowering, rather than empowering. Food, exercise, relationships, and meaningful work are all important components of wellness. But listening to the wrong messages about these areas of your life derails the pursuit of wellness, rather than supports it.

You are the expert at taking care of yourself. The doctor you see when your body is not working right is only one piece of your health. When it comes to health, people are used to being told what to do. I've had patients finally stop drinking because I told them to, though I doubt they did not already know drunkenness was a dangerous lifestyle. For some reason they needed the "expert" to say it.

You are the one who knows what is going on in your life. You are the one who knows what brings you joy and what stresses you out. You are the one who knows if you are lonely or tired or energized or filled with purpose or discouraged or excited out of your mind. No one else can look at your life and tell you five easy steps to health— and in only two easy weeks.

Cultural messages can be disempowering because they quickly steer us toward the negative. We fail when measured against those messages. We fail to have the body of the model in the ads. We fail to lift 180 pounds. We fail to stick to the diet that deprives us of our favorite foods. We fail to do as much as we think we should. We fail to attract as many Facebook friends as everyone else—or so we think.

Perhaps we're supposed to hear the messages and be inspired to achieve them. For some people that works. For many others— perhaps most others—failure is just one more thing to feel crummy about.

Blessing is a far more powerful motivator. A kind word from someone in a support group will do more for your overall wellness than a month of weights. Where are the blessings in your life? Who are the people who make you feel loved? Who are the ones who stand with you in suffering? What activities make you feel better for having done them—without regrets? Where do you find meaning in your life? How do you draw closer to God? Where do you find the connections that enrich your experience of body-and-spirit humanity?

No one can answer these questions for you, but these are the messages that will contribute to your health. Are you listening to your answers?

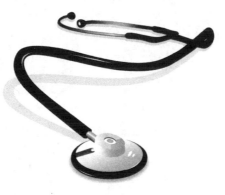

12

Don't Believe Everything
You Hear at Church

*If a church has to offer fried chicken to draw a crowd,
then something is wrong with the message.*

We might think that when the culture fails us with its messages that work against wellness, we can at least turn to the church. After all, the church connects us to God. The church is where we go when we are looking for more of God, our creator, who made us body-and-spirit. Unfortunately, the church carries false messages of its own that pull us away from health, rather than toward it.

Church fills you up. The filling station mentality is an endless problem. People go to church expecting to get filled up and tuned up for another week. They run their motors down during the week and go back for another filling.

That's not how life works, and church should not function that way. The church is there to help you figure out how to charge your battery every day of the week. Being a disciple of Jesus and experiencing God's presence in the here and now don't happen simply on Sundays. Expect the church to give you tools you can use all week, but the real experience of knowing God more deeply should happen Monday to Saturday as well as on Sunday. Too many churches foster a dependence on pastors and other paid staff to impart spiritual wisdom, rather than helping people to dig deeper with God in their real-life experience. The church ought to be helping people approach God without thinking they must have the help of a religious professional in order to do so. God fills you up, not the church, and God is open for business twenty-four hours a day. That simple shift in thinking can change your experience of God, which then touches every part of your life.

Change happens in an instant. Dramatic religious experiences are powerful. Conversion experiences, in particular, sometimes genuinely produce rapid change. The new believer puts the old ways behind and embraces new life in Christ. It's not always that way, though. Conversion often happens over a period of time. A deepening faith certainly happens over a period of time. We do people a disservice if we lead them to believe that a powerful experience changes everything in an instant. They wake up the morning after a retreat, and life is still there with all its mess and complications. We do not present a true understanding of the fullness of life when we set an expectation that everything will be sweetness and light in Jesus. If you have a powerful spiritual experience, embrace it. Savor it. Then let it change you and make you more whole over time.

Everybody knows the Bible. We make assumptions right and left at church about what people know about religion. Often these assumptions are dead wrong. We cannot assume that people read the Bible, or even that they own a Bible. They may not know the Bible stories church people refer to in casual conversation or sermons. For some people, just saying the name *Elijah* conjures up images of a massive fiery religious contest between the ancient Hebrews and the worshippers of Baal on top of Mount Carmel. But many others are quietly thinking, *Elijah who?* We bring about shame and guilt for people with our assumptions about what they should know. How can the church point people to wholeness they can find in God with that starting point? We can be a far more effective force of true change if we meet people where they are and lead them gently along the path of welcoming God into every part of their lives.

Being busy makes you more righteous. Despite theoretically advocating balance and priorities, the church does an incredible job of keeping people busy. We manage to make it sound like God's calling. How can you say no to a Bible study? How can you not serve on the committee when you are so gifted for the work? The sign-up list for the outreach team is in the foyer. God wants you to do this.

Life is a marathon, not a sprint. Churches burn out too many people with a sprint mentality. The rewards of a full and healthy life come from being able to sustain your efforts, even in your service to God.

We use volunteer physicians at the Church Health Center in addition to our paid staff doctors. Also, specialists who want to support our work agree to see patients we refer for free or low-cost care. But we purposely schedule volunteer doctors for only one shift every two or three months, and specialists for only two or three patients a month. At this pace, we have numerous doctors who stay with us for many, many years. We're asking them to run a well-paced marathon with us, not expend themselves with back-to-back sprints.

When churches keep people overly busy, they create time constraints that do not encourage exercise, relationships, reflection, nutritious meals, and other elements of a healthy lifestyle to sustain the whole person, not just the religious life. Pastors are often the most unhealthy people in the church because of the expectations they have for themselves and the expectations their congregations have for them. Being busy does not make you closer to God.

Fellowship trumps healthy eating. Often the least healthy meal we eat is at church. It's as if it's okay to eat all the chocolate cake you want because you're having fellowship over a meal. We create the idea of church as a cocoon from life. Somehow it's okay to set aside what we know about nutrition for the church potluck. It's acceptable to encourage indulgence in foods we don't eat otherwise because we're eating at church. I'm all for fellowship and the relationships that emerge from the church community, but church is not an escape from life. It ought to be what real life is. If a church has to offer fried chicken to draw a crowd, then something is wrong with the message.

Eight weeks is long enough. Churches are great at starting things and terrible at sustaining them. A visionary burst gets the ball rolling with some new ministry, and a few weeks of organizational flurry follow. Far too often, though, after six or eight weeks, the effort dies out. Leadership transitions. Participation dwindles. Meetings get canceled. People are on to the next new project.

Ted Turner, creator of the Cable News Network (CNN), pioneered a new frontier with twenty-four-hour news. Many doubted the effort was sustainable and asked how long he planned to stay on the air. He answered that he intended to stay on the air until the world ended. Then he would play "Nearer, My God, to Thee" and sign off.

Church programs and ministries don't have to last until the second coming of Christ. But it's harmful to launch new efforts we are not prepared to sustain. Ministries need a beginning, a middle, and an end, not a launch complete with fanfare and then a quiet disappearing act. In our work serving the poor at the Church Health Center, we've learned that it's better never to start something than to raise expectations and not follow through. Hope is a key component of wellness, and when we raise hope only to deliver disappointment, we are not helping people be healthier.

We don't talk about that. Churches are filled with people who have aging parents, and they're struggling to know how to care for them. Some of these parents have significant physical challenges or diseases like Alzheimer's. Others in the church duly ask, "How's your mother?" to which many people lie, "Mama's doing fine." The questioner may never get around to inquiring how the caregiver is doing. This goes on until Mama dies. At the funeral everybody says what a wonderful woman she was and what a great son or daughter you were. Then people tend to think they shouldn't talk about the loss, and it's as if the parent never lived. The truth is, people who suffer this kind of personal loss want to talk about Mama.

But we don't.

We could say the same thing about teen sexuality—or sexuality issues in general—or addictions, abuse, rebellious children, marital stresses, estranged siblings. We don't talk about those topics. Yet they are the messy stuff of life that happens even to Christians. How can we remind someone God is present in those situations when we don't want to be present in them ourselves? Churches have powerful opportunities to be places of healing if members would learn to talk lovingly about the experiences that assault the health of the whole person. Most churches don't do a good job of helping people wrestle through the tough challenges and reflect on how the experience impacts overall wellness.

You can't believe everything you hear in the culture on the subject of health, and churches don't always get it right, either. The pursuit of health sometimes feels like an uphill trek. But you are still the expert on you. It's your journey to wellness. Understanding messages gone awry can help you keep your eye on the goal of wellness rather than getting sidetracked by things you don't really believe. While you can't change everyone around you, you can make your personal choice to pursue health in your own life and to express wellness to others in your life.

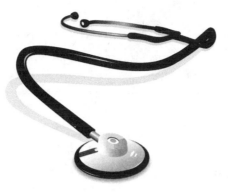

13

Prepare to Turn

Your mother doesn't work here. Clean up after yourself.

Every year thousands of college students take an art history class to fulfill a liberal arts requirement. They stare bleary-eyed at slide after slide of paintings that span the history of Western civilization and hope they remember the images long enough to pass the test.

And every now and then, something sticks.

In my one and only art history class, I encountered a particular Rembrandt painting that has spoken to me for decades. The painting is called *The Polish Rider*, and at first glance you might think it's just another medieval-looking rendition of a time and place foreign to most of us. A gallant, well-dressed young man, armed with a quiver of arrows and a sword, proudly sits astride a silvery white horse. A distant land beckons from the background. The horse is pulling toward the bend in the road that leads to that faraway place, but the young man turns and gazes at the place he is leaving.

Some art scholars, including my college professor, suggest this painting is an image of the prodigal son from Luke 15 in the New Testament. A wealthy man's cocky younger son demanded his inheritance while his father was still alive, and as soon as the money was in his hands, he left for a faraway place. Rembrandt perhaps captured, in medieval trappings, a moment of decision from this story. The young rider is in that split second when he could have realized the outrageous and destructive nature of his scheme and turned to go home to his father. The tug of the horse toward the road, though, tells us the man has already decided which direction he will go.

In all our lives, we experience that moment of decision. At the time, we may not realize the significance. Sometimes we miss the opportunity to take the turn that leads to wellness, just as the prodigal son missed his opportunity to turn back to the love of his father.

Turn toward wellness.

Years ago, Rob attended Rhodes College in Memphis. A straight-A student, he was popular, thoughtful, and involved in various social programs. Rob gravitated toward the Church Health Center, and he and I began playing racquetball together every week. Rob received a scholarship through the National Health Services Corporation for medical school. He chose to attend the Armed Services Medical School in Bethesda, Maryland, not because he was interested in the military, but because the school offered the chance to study on Native American reservations and in other underserved areas of the country.

While he was in medical school, Rob sent me long typed letters about what he was learning and how he was becoming involved with the homeless in Washington, D.C. Joyously, he also fell in love with a young woman in her second year of medical school. Tragically, at the end of Rob's third year, his girlfriend was killed in a traffic accident. Rob was devastated, and I didn't hear from him for a long time. Eventually, though, he seemed to get back on track. Then, after months of planning that no one was aware of, Rob killed himself. He left a note that ended with, "I am the ray of sunshine through the trees, the birdsong in the forest rain after drought, the warm feeling of love. Now and then, think of me and smile."

Rob had amazing compassion in his heart, but he couldn't see his way through his loss or allow others to carry him through the tragedy. Though he cared deeply about alleviating other people's hardships, he didn't make the turn toward wholeness for himself.

Joseph lived through the horrors of the Bosnian War in the early 1990s, including ten months in a concentration camp. When I asked Joseph why he was put in the camp, he gave a weak laugh and said, "Because I was Bosnian." After the war, Joseph left the chaotic region and came to Memphis. Over the next two years, he brought other members of his family to the United States. Joseph and his wife were both students at the University of Memphis, Joseph worked at FedEx, and together they looked forward to their futures. His mother, Yanni, however, could not find a way to make Memphis her home. She frequently relived the horror of the war and desperately ached for the friends and family she left behind. Yanni cried for long stretches of the day, and antidepressant medications did not seem to help.

Yanni and Joseph came through the same war, the same shredding of the fabric of their lives. No one could take back the war or put people's lives back together just the way they were before. The difference was Joseph took a turn that Yanni never did. Joseph turned toward joy and wholeness and life, but Yanni couldn't do it.

Old habits die hard.

The easiest route is to keep going with old habits. That does not require turning or making a decision. We can simply trot the horse right through those life intersections that offer us the opportunity to turn and take a new path. After a while we may never even notice the crossroads, much less realize that we are capable of making a choice. Life is what it is, and as miserable as it seems at times, we settle into it.

The problem with staying on the same road is that we fall into the same potholes again and again. We expend the same energy climbing out of the same holes, and we are no farther along on the road to anywhere. We lose sight of the fact that there even is an "anywhere" beyond the rim of the pothole we spend our lives falling into and climbing out of. And the more we do this, the more rutted the habit becomes and the less likely we are to break out of patterns that are far from healthy.

Jesus' followers took the turn. And the next turn. And the next turn. Jesus stood on the shore of the Sea of Galilee and called Peter and Andrew and James and John, two sets of fisherman brothers. "Come, follow me," he said. They had a thriving business and families—not such a bad life. But when Jesus invited them to look down a different road, they took the turn. Matthew was busy counting his Roman coins and sorting out how much he had to fork over to the government for the taxes he collected and how much he could stockpile for himself. When Jesus said, "Follow me," Matthew got up and left the tax business. Philip got excited about Jesus, and he raced off to find Nathanael. Nathanael was more skeptical of this "new road," but he agreed to at least scope it out. Jesus met him there on the road and was quite persuasive. Nathanael took the turn.

Eventually Jesus had twelve people who became his closest followers, the disciples. Each one took a turn from the safe life he knew into a relationship with Jesus that would lead into the unknown. Together these twelve became a community, and together they took a turn toward the kingdom of God. They didn't always get what Jesus talked about. They didn't always listen very well. They sometimes heard what they wanted to hear instead of what Jesus said. But they faithfully traipsed around the countryside with him for three years.

Another young man came to Jesus with questions about how he could participate in the kingdom of God and have the abundant life Jesus talked so much about. After some back-and-forth conversation to get to the heart of the question, Jesus said, "Go, sell your possessions and give to the poor, and you will have treasure in heaven. Then come, follow me" (Matthew 19:21). Jesus pointed to a turn in the road, but the young man couldn't make the turn. He walked away. He was a wealthy person, and he couldn't let go and choose what he could not be sure of.

When Jesus died—something Jesus' followers didn't expect despite all the preparation Jesus gave them—most of the disciples scattered in fear. But they regrouped, and once again Jesus came to them where they were. This time they gathered in a locked room to try to figure out what came next. Jesus, raised from the dead, showed up, and the disciples took yet another turn to give their lives to something brand new—being witnesses to the power and presence of Christ in the world. They were on the journey together, and the church was born.

Meet yourself where you are.

A young man's wealth is certainly not the only obstacle that gets in the way of taking the turn in the road toward health. Sometimes the reasons run deep. For instance, 90 percent of women who are morbidly obese have been sexually abused. From their youth they have heard messages that say they are less than valuable and have been shamed into believing that, and the effect shows up in their weight. For them, the real question is not, "How can I lose a hundred pounds in the next ninety days?" That would not solve the problem. It would not make them whole.

Dysfunctional family patterns run deep. Relationships profoundly disappoint us. Careers stall or disintegrate. Trauma turns life inside out. Ingrained comforting habits rise to the surface and we take the familiar road even though we know it's full of potholes. Wellness starts in recognizing and naming the forces that keep us on the familiar road, afraid of taking a turn.

We must meet ourselves where we are. Paying far too much attention to the standards other people set, we fall short and then feel judged for falling short. It hurts, and we know it hurts. We even judge ourselves. Nevertheless, we keep walking around in shoes that pinch our feet with every step. Change begins in meeting yourself where you are, admitting what hurts, and deciding to take the turn that only you can take. Years ago I made up some rules by which the Church Health Center would operate, and one of them was, "Your mother doesn't work here. Clean up after yourself." No one else can change your level of wellness. You have to do that for yourself.

Sometimes change comes suddenly and may be outside of your control. This happened to Yanni when the war in Bosnia blew up her life. Life as you know it may blow up relationally, economically, and physically for many reasons beyond your control. Sometimes change through life circumstances is gentler, even unnoticeable as it happens. Every night you read with your son, then one night he is engrossed in a book on his own, and you start a new season. One day you're wiping faces, and the next, it seems, you're leaving your kids at the college dorm. You see your reflection in a store window and think, *That person looks just like me but twenty pounds heavier and with gray hair.*

You can't undo the explosions. You can't freeze-frame stages of life. But neither do you have to be passive about taking the turns of life. Change does not have to be something that happens to you. It can be something you step into and embrace and freely choose. When it comes to your overall health—your sense of wholeness as a body-and-spirit being created and loved by God—you can choose change.

Change you choose begins in a moment of awareness that

another road exists. The idea may take some getting used to before you're ready to follow the fork in the road, and then it will take even more time to discover what awaits you on the new journey. For a while you may think often of the old familiar road, or even imagine yourself back on it. Gradually, though, you begin to notice and appreciate the new scenery, and the new road feels like the road you should have been on all along.

The prodigal son had his heart set on one road. Perhaps he had been dreaming of leaving home for years, until he could not stand the thought of staying there one more minute waiting for his inheritance. So he hurtled himself down the road to a faraway country. As he traveled the road, though, he discovered it was toxic. He was not happier or more full of joy. Money created more problems than it solved. In the end, he was alone and humiliated. At last, standing penniless in a pigpen, he remembered his father and the place where he had known love. He was ready to make a turn and go home.

When the father saw his son coming, he rejoiced. He welcomed him. He loved him. He threw a party. His son was home!

Whether or not *The Polish Rider* is an image of the prodigal son, Rembrandt painted a masterpiece called *The Return of the Prodigal Son*. Equally medieval, the tattered, exhausted younger son collapses into his father's welcoming arms in a decisive moment of surrender to his father's love. What a picture of the way God receives us when we turn toward God's love in our lives. The culture is full of messages that pull us away from joy and wholeness. Churches get in ruts that undermine true health. New roads are scary. But the heart of God is constant.

Don't miss the intersection that can put you on the path to the kind of wellness God has in mind for you. You can choose change. You can choose health care you can live with.

Prepare to turn.

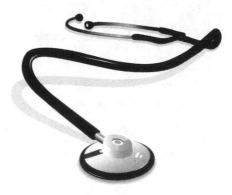

14

Treat Yourself the Way
You Want Others to Treat You

Things that seem impossible to us are possible to God.

W hen I was in medical school, the pull away from the life of the spirit was so intense that I regularly sought ways to keep myself grounded in faith. When I was reading the Bible one day, the beauty of Paul's words in Colossians 3 gripped me in a fresh way.

Paul spent three years in Ephesus, about a hundred miles west of Colosse. A man named Epaphras learned the gospel from Paul and carried it to Colosse. So Paul was sort of the grandfather of the church there. Years later, when Paul was a prisoner in Rome, he wrote to the Colossians because false teachers were scrambling up the theological landscape and Paul wanted to set matters straight. Christ comes first in all things, plain and simple. Christ shows us God. Christ *is* God. Through Christ, God gives us new life, so we should step into the new wardrobe that God gives us to wear in this new life.

I began to read these verses from Colossians 3 every day, a habit I have maintained for decades.

Therefore, as God's chosen people, holy and dearly loved, clothe yourselves with compassion, kindness, humility, gentleness and patience. Bear with each other and forgive whatever grievances you may have against one another. Forgive as the Lord forgave you. And over all these virtues put on love, which binds them all together in perfect unity. (Colossians 3:12–14)

We put on the clothes God gives us.

This passage is about how believers are to treat one another. It's not about how I see myself in isolation, apart from other people. It's not primarily about how I can get my own life in order and get right with God to find personal salvation. Rather, these words speak to how we live in the here and now with the problems that happen in the broken world and broken lives. The characteristics—the clothes God gives us and wants us to put on—are a picture of healthy relational living. As we get comfortable wearing these clothes, we get closer and closer to God and show each other the wholeness God wants for us.

Paul calls his readers "God's chosen people, holy and dearly loved." That's the starting point for how we relate to each other. God loves us. God chooses us. God forms us into a community. In community we share an experience of God at work in us to make us holy—more and more like God—and revel in God's love in every dimension of our lives. We don't scrounge up all these great qualities with our own efforts. They begin in our relationship with God and reflect the way God relates to us.

Compassion.

Kindness.

Humility.

Gentleness.

Patience.

Forgiveness.

Love.

These are not always easy traits, so I'm not going to suggest they are. The list of reasons why we fall short of treating each other this way is long. But these are the garments God asks us to wear as we relate to each other.

When Church Health Center Wellness first opened, we camped on James 5:14, "Is any one of you sick? He should call the elders of the church to pray over him and anoint him with oil in the name of the Lord." Through the years of our ministry, however, Colossians 3:12–14 has come to the forefront more and more. We call these pieces of clothing God gives us "the virtues," and they have become the heart of what we do at the Wellness center. Everything we plan and implement touches on one of the virtues at some level. Whether we're running exercise programs, cancer support groups, nutrition classes, or personal counseling, we want to see the virtues play out in as many ways as possible. If an idea comes up for a new program or service we might offer, our first question is, "How does this touch on the virtues?" If we can't answer that question, we don't do it.

The architect of the Wellness building had the concept of developing public art pieces all inspired by these verses from Colossians 3. Artists all over the country contributed. The goal was that these virtues be not just an intellectual concept, but a reality people encounter as they're exercising, eating, swimming, and so on. Through art, we engage people in the virtues. If you are hanging on to the side of the pool because of pain, the tiles under your nose are words of comfort and hope. When you're exercising, you see fabric art hanging from the ceiling. The virtues literally are right over your head.

Several years ago we added some funky art to the front of our medical clinic. Each tower features a different virtue. The art is a combination of metal and glass, but within the glass is the virtue in a dozen different languages. These virtues translate across languages, and clothing ourselves with them envelops the world in the power of the gospel. Now we see these virtues as the subject for daily meditation.

Through our work, we're building a community of wellness that encourages people to engage with these virtues in the ways they relate to each other. Clothing yourself with these virtues leads to what the fullness of life is all about—being a whole, healthy person in relationship with God. It's not as if we can single out just one virtue. They come as a set, a wardrobe ensemble. To be fully dressed, we must put on all of them.

How do you treat yourself?

The community factor is only one dimension of the virtues, however. We've seen some of the most powerful demonstrations of the virtues in the way people have learned to treat themselves.

We understand what it means to treat someone else with compassion, but do we understand what it means to treat ourselves with compassion?

To treat ourselves with kindness? Humility? Gentleness? Patience? Forgiveness? Love?

The inability to treat ourselves with these virtues is a huge obstacle to seeing ourselves as the whole people God wants us to be. It is surprisingly easy to convince ourselves we don't deserve to treat ourselves the way we hope others would treat us.

In the world of education, Howard Gardner, a professor at Harvard, is well known for his theory of multiple intelligences. Traditional IQ tests do a good job of measuring logical or linguistic intelligence, but there are lots of ways to be smart that these tests don't capture. One of the intelligences is "intrapersonal"—in other words, how well you know yourself. Self-smart. A person with intrapersonal intelligence has a good understanding of personal strengths, what makes the person unique and how the person might respond in emotions and actions to various situations. But not everybody is equally self-smart, any more than everybody is equally music smart, or logic smart. Some people have more natural aptitude than others, but we can all learn.

I wonder if we would be able to treat ourselves with the virtues of Colossians 3 if we had a better understanding of what it means to be self-smart, and if we valued it more. We might see more clearly what trips us up and makes us stumble in our pursuit of wellness. And if we better understand what makes us stumble, we might be able to respond with compassion, humility, kindness, gentleness, patience, forgiveness, and love toward ourselves.

We need to put on these virtues every day. It's a daily commitment, a constant reworking in our lives and relationships. The experience changes as the circumstances of life change.

These virtues are the context in which real change happens. They are not only how we relate to each other and invite God's healing into relationships, but also how we must relate to ourselves and invite God's healing into the places where our own lives are broken.

If compassion is an expression of care and the desire to help, in what ways are you overlooking caring for yourself?

If kindness is a sympathetic attitude with the willingness to be helpful whenever possible, how can you be sympathetic and helpful to yourself?

If humility is the willingness to give up something that should rightfully be yours, in what areas of your life do you need to give something up—to help yourself?

If gentleness is choosing a mild disposition rather than using force, what do you need to stop beating yourself up about?

If patience is the ability to undergo problems or opposition without complaining, what do you need to give yourself some time and space for as you begin to make changes?

If forgiveness is letting go of being wronged, how do you need to let go of wronging yourself?

If love ultimately is seeing in yourself the intrinsic value that God sees in you, what do you need to move out of the way of that picture?

These virtues are the setting in which we move toward wellness in body-and-spirit. They begin in God and they drive us closer to God. They help us experience God's presence in the here and now. Things that seem impossible to us are possible to God, and God reminds us of that in this model of how we relate to each other.

We cannot truly be well without the virtues. They are fundamental to understanding how we are connected to God and how God wants us to be connected to each other.

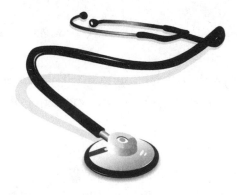

15

Put On Compassion

*If an act of true compassion doesn't bring a tear to your eye,
you have to question your sense of humanity.*

Chastity was eight years old and her family's translator. She was in the clinic at the Church Health Center with her Spanish-speaking mother and baby sister. The baby had a simple cold and I assured the mother, through Chastity, that she would be fine. Then Chastity explained that she herself had a stomachache. After a couple of minutes of conversation, I was sure something was not right with this story.

"Where are you living?" I asked Chastity.

"In a homeless shelter," she answered.

"How did you come to be living there?"

"Our daddy found somebody else," she said, "and he doesn't love us anymore."

It was pretty clear why her stomach hurt, and I didn't have any medicine for that.

But I could make a phone call to the pastor of a Hispanic church a few miles from the clinic. Before the sun was down that day, Chastity and her mother and baby sister were out of the shelter and in the arms of a congregation that embraced them and made them their own. Nobody can make Chastity's father love her, but the church family brought goodness into Chastity's life, and things are better.

That's compassion.

Annie was seventy-four and very pleasant, but didn't know the time of day. She could perform a few basic activities of daily living, but she depended almost entirely on "Sister Penny," a woman her own age whose only relationship to Annie was that they attended the same church for forty years. Five years earlier, Annie began showing signs of dementia, and Penny started to look after her.

"Who else is going to do it?" Penny asked matter-of-factly.

That's compassion.

Bessie was ninety-four and living alternately with two nieces in their fifties. I asked one day, "How is it that it fell to the two of you to care for her?"

They nearly tripped over each other to answer. One said, "Bessie was always around while we were growing up. I don't know what we would have done without her." The other added, "When our mother died, almost her last words to us were, 'Don't forget about Bessie.' So she's been with us ever since."

The task was getting harder as Bessie was less able to care for herself, but clearly looking after her was a labor of love.

That's compassion.

Hospitality is the heart of compassion.

Compassion is not just being nice to strangers. It goes beyond writing a check to an organization working on the front lines of poverty, as valuable as that is. It's not the same as feeling sorry that someone you know is having a tough time. It certainly is not the same as saying, "I'll be praying for you."

When we look at the compassion of Jesus, we notice a thread of hospitality running through his encounters. Jesus was on the move most of the time during his three-year earthly ministry. He didn't have a sprawling house with guest rooms and matching dishes, but he was hospitable wherever he went. He attended a wedding in Cana as a guest and ended up providing the wine, which was the role of the host. When the hillside crowds were hungry and Jesus' disciples were ready to send them away and be done with it, he had compassion and hosted a dinner for more than five thousand people.

Jesus shared meals with the scum of society—Jewish tax collectors who worked for the hated Roman government. Jesus called a tax collector, Matthew, to his inner circle and openly ate dinner at his house, while the Jewish religious leaders of the day asked, "Why does your teacher eat with tax collectors and 'sinners'?" (Matthew 9:11), as if nothing could be more disgusting. He called Zacchaeus out of the sycamore tree, where Zacchaeus had perched to watch Jesus go by in the crowded Jericho street, and invited himself to the tax collector's house.

People with leprosy—which likely covered a range of skin diseases—were forced to live on the outskirts of town, away from their families, in an attempt to contain the spread of the disease. Nobody in their right mind touched a person with leprosy. But Jesus did. When a man with leprosy came to him for healing, Jesus touched him. He welcomed the interaction with a man most people kept their distance from.

Jesus talked to women and blessed children in a time and place where women and children barely ranked above property. When a Roman centurion asked for healing for his servant, Jesus got up and went to the servant. Over and over again, Jesus made room in his life for people who didn't fit. He didn't take a writing retreat to record some great story ideas; he told stories among the people. He listened. He touched. He inconvenienced himself. He brought healing to people the society bigwigs tended to write off. He welcomed the rejected. He was hospitable, and out of his hospitality flowed the kingdom of God.

When we begin to understand hospitality, then we begin to understand compassion. Most people don't appreciate the depth of this word, *compassion*. Hospitality says, "Others may want nothing to do with you, but I welcome you into my space." And when we actively welcome, we reach out and touch. We become compassionate and behave in compassionate ways toward real people who may be on the outskirts of our lives or our society.

Compassion is an intense desire to embrace people in a way that is not the norm in our world today. Through this embracing, we show what the kingdom of God is all about. That means making room in our lives for people who might not be there now. It means being hospitable toward people who are different from us and choosing to welcome them into our lives. I don't mean making room in the sense of scooting over to make just barely enough space to squeeze one more person in a crowded row. That is neither hospitality nor compassion. Rather, I'm talking about an intentional attitude of welcome toward the people God puts in our lives—whether immigrant families, old aunts, or perfect strangers.

Compassion is unselfish. It allows another person into your world and gives you the opportunity to offer whatever you have to give—without weighing the cost or secretly hoping for something in return. Compassion acts in a way that is completely unexpected and thoroughly motivated by love. It's a moving experience at every turn. I don't find it particularly common. As much as we might think it's a nice idea, we don't experience or extend compassion every day. But when compassion happens, everyone involved—whether on the giving or receiving end—is better because of it. If an act of true compassion doesn't bring a tear to your eye, you have to question your sense of humanity.

Treat yourself with compassion.

God made room for you. In sending Jesus into body-and-spirit humanity, God reached out to be connected to you. God welcomed you in from the outskirts and gave you a place to belong in the kingdom of God. In compassionate mercy, you were made part of God's family!

As you continue to discover what wellness means in your own life, ask how you can put on compassion toward others and yourself. Being compassionate toward others might actually be the easier task. Once you start looking, you will see needs you can respond to, people you can welcome into your life without expecting anything from them, opportunities to give, ways to open your heart and invite others into your space.

You might have to dig a little deeper to understand how to show compassion toward yourself. How might you be rejecting yourself because, for some reason, you think you don't deserve compassion? How might you be turning your back on your own value as a body-and-spirit being created and loved by God? How might you be leaving yourself standing on the outskirts of God's kingdom, waiting for a place to belong?

Look at yourself through the same eyes of welcoming love through which God sees you. See the wholeness God wants for you, body-and-spirit. If God wants it for you, shouldn't you want it for yourself?

I had a patient I called the "nickel lady." She lived on only about $200 a month from Social Security, but she kept a stack of nickels that she gave to the Church Health Center. Every day she added a nickel to the stack. Whenever she came in to see us, she brought her nickels as a donation. She believed in the value of what we do not just for her, but even more for others who need the care we provide. The nickel lady didn't have much to begin with, but she gave what she had, and she made a habit of it.

Starting small adds up. Even small habits bring big changes when it comes to health. Make sure to put a nickel in the compassion stack every day. It will be good for your health.

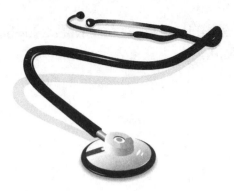

16

Put On Kindness

Don't judge. Just help.

When Hurricane Katrina slammed the Louisiana coast in 2005 and demolished New Orleans, ten thousand people deluged Memphis in a matter of days. An incredible percentage of these people were uninsured, and many overwhelmed us at the Church Health Center. We weren't prepared. How could we be? People with diabetes left Louisiana with no insulin and others abandoned anti-seizure medications as they fled for their lives. No doctors—if they could be found—would call in prescriptions to Memphis. And people showed up at our doors addicted to drugs and abruptly without their dealers. Now they were in Memphis going through sudden withdrawal and looking for narcotics.

The response from the people of Memphis was amazing. No one was fooled; addicts were trying to avoid a forced withdrawal, and under other circumstances we would have turned away the narcotics seekers. But at that moment, when the infrastructure of their lives imploded and washed into the ocean, the addicts didn't need judgment that forced them into withdrawal. The decision to treat them had nothing to do with approving of substance abuse. Doctors and nurses and volunteers stepped up with kindness that relieved suffering. A week's worth of narcotics could get people through the worst part of realizing that a hurricane literally had blown through their lives. Maybe in a week they would be willing to deal with the substance abuse problem as they faced the reality of trying to rebuild their lives in a new city. Or maybe in a week they would have found a new supplier in Memphis. Either way, from the point of view of the virtues of Colossians 3, I had no doubt that the right decision was to offer these patients the same quality of care we offered to all our patients.

Don't judge. Just help. That's kindness.

A few years ago, a couple of Jehovah's Witnesses brought a young woman to the clinic. She was only seventeen, and they were worried about her. They met her through doing what Jehovah's Witnesses do—going up and down the street knocking on doors and trying to engage people in conversation. She would talk to them at the door, and after a series of visits, they learned her story. She was from Liberia and lived through the Liberian Civil War, a horror that conscripted children and trained them to kill. A band of child soldiers came through her village and slaughtered practically everybody. They dragged her parents and siblings out of the house and killed them. The girl survived by huddling under a couple of sofa cushions in a closet, and miraculously they did not find her. For more than a week, she ate the insides of the cushions. She went to live in a refugee camp, and from there, someone sponsored her to come to the United States. She was staying with a long-lost relative who didn't pay much attention to her, but at least she had a place to live.

The Jehovah's Witnesses brought her to the clinic because they figured out she had an unnatural craving to eat sponges. Whenever they asked if they could help her in any way, she wanted sponges.

I pointed out that the sponges were comfort food. She turned to sponges when she felt stressed because sponge cushions saved her life. Whatever you think of the theology of the Jehovah's Witnesses, they took this young woman under their wings and cared for her. Anyone willing to care for somebody others would regard as an outcast is okay by me.

Don't judge. Just help. That's kindness.

Marsha spent half her life in and out of doctors' offices. At the age of fifteen, she developed insulin-dependent diabetes. In her early twenties, she married and had a daughter, Carrie. When Marsha was twenty-eight, she had her first heart attack and a bypass operation. Her diabetes continued to worsen. With every step she took, Marsha was in pain. She was thirty-three when she first came to the Church Health Center. Her job was in danger because she missed so much work due to her declining health. She was on ten different medications she could not afford, and now her eight-year-old daughter had diabetes as well. Her husband had long since left and never sent a penny of support.

One day she came for an unscheduled visit and started to sob uncontrollably. Nothing I did comforted her. "Marsha," I tried to say gently, "what's wrong?"

Through the tears she told the story. "Carrie got sick over the weekend and I could not get hold of her doctor, so I took her to the minor medical clinic. They said she had bronchitis and gave me a prescription. But I paid all the money I had to the doctor's office. I had the prescription but no money to pay for it." By this point tears streamed down her face. "Can you imagine what it feels like to know your child is sick and there is a way to make her feel better, but there is nothing you can do?"

I reached out and put my arm around Marsha. "You know, we see children here."

For some reason this had never occurred to Marsha. "You mean

I can bring Carrie here?"

So Carrie became our patient, too. Marsha's vascular disease progressed until one night, at the age of forty-one, she went to sleep and did not wake up. By now Carrie was sixteen. I met Carrie's father at the funeral. He promised he would look out for his daughter, but he never did, so she lived with her grandmother.

This is when Debbie, a nurse at the Church Health Center, stepped into Carrie's life in a way that is almost beyond kindness. It began by helping Carrie get a dress for a school dance. Then Debbie started to include Carrie in her own family's events, including a trip to Washington, D.C., to see her husband's parents. Debbie and her husband, Butch, helped Carrie apply for a scholarship to go to college and made sure she got there. When Carrie developed an irregular heart rhythm, most likely related to her diabetes, Debbie and Butch were there with her in the hospital.

It would be easy to focus on the tragedy of Marsha's and Carrie's lives, but as the saga unfolded over a period of time, the deeper meaning for me was the unbounded kindness that Debbie expressed to Carrie over and over. As Debbie put it, "I just want to make sure she knows she is loved." What an unbelievable gift to give someone else's daughter.

Don't judge. Just help. That's kindness.

Kindness begins in God.

"Kindness" in the Bible is one of the most frequent descriptions of God. Old Testament writers speak of the abundance of God's goodness to the people of God. In the Psalms, worshippers see God as always ready with mercy and help and don't hesitate to call on God. The prophets, who spoke God's word to the people even when it wasn't pretty, show us that the kindness of God is all the more amazing against the backdrop of the chronic sin of the people. In the New Testament, Paul reminds us that God's kindness leads us to repentance—and into relationship with God, where we experience God's kindness toward us over and over and over.

In the course of the entire Bible, we see that God consistently connects with people in kindness, and not because they deserve it. God is in it for the long haul. Kindness is not one isolated deed. It's not just a moment. It's a way of relating to people. Most of us are not able to do this out of instinct. When you're behind the wheel of a car and someone pulls out in front of you, kindness is not your first impulse. When you're with another person, working or living together day in and day out, responding with kindness is not always easy. We leap to judgments instead—reasons why the person does not deserve our kindness.

If God kept a list of why we don't deserve kindness, where would we be? In many ways, kindness is a learned response that comes from choosing it and practicing it, even when people do stupid things. When things don't go well, the ability to respond to another person with tenderness requires enormous discipline.

Don't judge. Just help.

And when we do have an impulse toward kindness, how easy is it to talk ourselves out of following it? We sense someone needs to talk, but we remember our own lengthy to-do list. We think a grieving family could use a hot meal, but we tell ourselves we don't have time to cook one. A sincere compliment crosses our minds but never passes our lips. Before we know it, rather than being a virtue that characterizes the way we live, kindness becomes a chore we have to schedule. We all get busy, but when we're too busy to enjoy doing good deeds, too busy to *be* a kind person, we damage our own health as well as the health of those around us.

Kindness reflects our experience of God's kindness toward us and connects us with each other. I never know what I'm going to see when I walk into an exam room. What a moment of grace it is when I open the door and can sense that the patient does not have an agenda to push or demands to make on me or anyone else in the clinic. Even though the patient may be ill, the attitude is not "What can I get from you?" but "Here I am, just doing whatever I can to be faithful to the love God shows me." Patients like this are so grateful for the love they feel God has for them that they treat me and everyone else with the same kindness. I leave the encounter enriched every time.

Treat yourself with kindness.

We can be pretty good at beating ourselves up.

"I shouldn't have done that."

"I should have said this."

"Why did I eat that cake? I'm an idiot."

"I can't quit smoking. I'm a weak person."

"I'm just not smart enough."

"No one will hire me. I'm worthless."

The things you say to yourself, whether out loud or in your head, can be some of the harshest judgments you ever endure. Does that give you joy? Does that point you to God? Does that take you deeper into God's kingdom?

Treat yourself with kindness. Point out the positive in yourself. Recognize it's not a sin if you need a nap. Accept help if someone offers. Give yourself a pep talk when you need it, not a lecture. When you disappoint yourself, help yourself get up and try again. Be kind to yourself for no other reason than because God loves you. It will be good for your health.

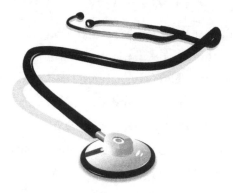

17

Put On Humility

Working on humility is a daily experience.

Y ou have AIDS." I was certain of it or I wouldn't have said it. This was years ago, when medications for AIDS were in their infancy.

Ron denied it. It just wasn't possible. But I was sure, and reluctantly my patient agreed to the blood test that would confirm. And it did.

"The good news," I told Ron, "is that you have treatment possibilities." Drugs for AIDS were new and incredibly expensive, so the Church Health Center did not have them. However, an Adult Special Care Clinic at the hospital could help him.

He refused to go.

"Why not?" I wanted to know.

"I know I would have acquired AIDS before I became a Christian," he explained. "I did drugs in those days, but it's all in the past. Now I'm a DJ on a Christian radio station. My friends only know who I am today. If I go to the clinic, people will recognize me and figure out I'm living a lie. I can't go."

Ron kept coming to see me, but I could not do a lot for him.

The clinic where he could get help remained out of the question. When people noticed that he lost a lot of weight and was quite sick, he told them he had cancer.

"You have cancer of the soul," I said at one point. I didn't see him for a while after that conversation.

Then one night in the middle of winter, I got a phone call from his mother. She said he was dying and the only person he wanted to talk to was me. Would I come?

This man lived in Hurt Village, one of the most economically depressed housing projects in Memphis. It was not a place where I needed to show my white face at night. Fortunately, Stan, an African American medical assistant, offered to go with me. So we went. It was dark, and I was still wearing the white coat that identified me as a doctor. Having Stan with me helped to quell some trepidation, but it was scary nevertheless. Shadows shrouded the apartment building, except for a bunch of people standing outside one door.

We found the right apartment, and the man's mother expressed sincere gratitude that we had come. She had no idea why he wanted to talk to me, but he kept insisting. They had run out of money a long time ago. With an unpaid electric bill, they had no heat and no light. A couple of candles flickered as my eyes adjusted to the interior gloom and I saw Ron lying on the couch. The smell of death hung in the room.

Ron motioned for me to come closer, so I knelt by the couch and leaned over his face. Talking took great effort for him, but he was determined.

"Do you think God can forgive me for what I've done?" he asked.

"Yes, I think so."

"Do you really think so?"

"Yes."

That was the extent of our conversation. I was Ron's doctor, and in that moment when death loomed, I was his pastor.

The next day his mother called to tell me Ron died during the night. I ran into his wife some time later at a church where I spoke. In my conversations with both his mother and wife, it was clear they thought he died from cancer. He never told a soul the truth.

What a terrible load for anyone to carry, and what an awful way to die. If this man had just been able to understand the power of humility, he could have had what he needed most during that season of his life—a community that embraced him, forgave the early mistakes, and assured him of God's love. The inability to humble himself meant he died without these comforts.

A little humility goes a long way.

Humility is elusive. Many people see it as a false virtue. Can you set out to be humbler? Wouldn't that mean you somehow take pride in being humble?

People also see humility as a sign of weakness, rather than a positive trait. Humility does not mean you don't stand up for yourself when it's the right thing to do. It doesn't mean you lie down and invite people to run over you. It doesn't mean you are weak. It certainly does not mean you don't stand up for other people who are suffering or oppressed.

Humility is a sign of strength. It means you do not first think about yourself at every turn. It means you don't become consumed with what you need before you think about what someone else needs. Humility says, "I care about my neighbor, and I am strong enough to put my neighbor's needs first before I take care of myself."

Every passenger on every plane hears the flight attendant say that in the event of a loss of cabin pressure, oxygen masks will drop from the panels above the seats. Passengers traveling with someone who requires assistance should put on their own masks first, then provide assistance. The airlines say this because people often have the instinct to help the other person first. In such a moment, it seems right to care for the people who can't care for themselves in that particular task. Perhaps this is a God-given instinct toward humility.

Unfortunately, we don't see this instinct in most situations. If it's not an emergency—and perhaps even if it is—we easily pass over the person who has no advocate in the situation, no voice in the circumstance. To care for these people, we have to be willing to sit on our own egos and say, "I'm not what matters most here."

Pride is the American way. We obsess over being able to tell people what we've accomplished and what we're sure we can do. How often do we miss what someone else says because our minds are already racing ahead to what we're going to say in response? We don't let ourselves truly hear what the other person is saying because the unwritten goal is not to learn something from the conversation, but rather to make ourselves the topic of the conversation and prove our own value.

Pride leads us to block people from having a place in our lives. Lovesick teenagers pine for affection from one person and look right past others who would be willing and able to give the love they need. We set up false standards, and when people don't measure up, we don't give them any place in our lives. We turn our backs on friendship and expressions of care because of some crazy prideful notion of who is worthy to care for us.

The Old Testament tells the story of Naaman, an Aramean army commander who stood on his accomplishment of military victories. He was a valiant soldier, and everybody knew it. The king of Aram was the president of Naaman's fan club. But Naaman had an aggravating skin disease he couldn't get rid of.

A young servant girl from Israel, who had been captured by the Aramean army, suggested that Naaman should go see Elisha, the prophet of Israel. It seemed like a long shot—what could a servant girl possibly know?—but Naaman went. And he took gifts—lots of money and high-end clothing. He would pay any price to be healed.

When Naaman arrived at Elisha's door, Elisha didn't even get out of his easy chair. He sent a message. "Go, wash yourself seven times in the Jordan, and your flesh will be restored and you will be cleansed" (2 Kings 5:10).

Naaman was indignant. How dare he not even come out and see me? How dare he send me to some filthy river? I can do better than the Jordan, of all places.

Once again the servants went into action. Was it really so hard to go dip in the Jordan? Just try it.

Naaman finally set aside his own sense of accomplishment and listened to the seemingly inconsequential people in his life. He went down to the Jordan and counted off seven dips—and the leprosy disappeared. A little humility went a long way in the life of Naaman.

Working on humility is a daily experience. I know very few truly humble people, but I have enormous respect for the ones I know.

Debbie Fields, the Mrs. Fields behind the cookie empire, supports our work at the Church Health Center. She called me one day to say she was at the FedEx Forum, the sports arena in Memphis, and the woman running the elevator had the most disgusting, disfiguring growth hanging off her face. Could I help?

I thought it would be no big deal, but the condition was truly severe. The woman had an incredible personality, but knowing what her own face looked like—and how it put people off—made her withdrawn. I was glad to arrange for the woman to see John, a dermatologist who had once been a clinic assistant at the Church Health Center. Over a period of several months, he was able to make things much better for this woman. Debbie followed the case, even offering to pay for John's services. When he refused payment, Debbie responded by baking him a batch of chocolate chip cookies in her own oven.

Mrs. Fields certainly could hold her own against Naaman in a things-to-be-proud-of contest. No doubt she had other things to do than notice the person operating the elevator. But she could see past her own considerable accomplishments and into the need in someone else's life. (And now I tell my clinic assistants that if they work hard, someday Mrs. Fields may bake them cookies!)

Mrs. Thomas came to me to get her toenails cut. She had an active mind in her later years, but limited physical mobility. She couldn't bend down, and her toenails had thickened from a fungus. Every few months, I cut them. It took all my strength—and clippings were likely to shoot off like missiles. Cutting her nails was always a humbling experience. I've heard other doctors say, "I don't do feet," but I always try to remember that Jesus washed the feet of the disciples.

About fifteen years ago I happened on the story of a Russian peasant who wanted to understand what it meant to pray without ceasing. He met an elderly spiritual guide who introduced him to the "Jesus Prayer," which goes back at least to the sixth century in the Eastern Orthodox tradition of Christianity. The Jesus Prayer says simply, "Jesus, Son of God, have mercy on me, a sinner." For centuries Christians have prayed this prayer repeatedly as a way of being present and in relationship with God throughout the day. I probably repeat it ten thousand times a day. It's always right there under my breath, behind my thoughts, reminding me who Jesus is and who I am, and my desperate, humble need for him.

Treat yourself with humility.

Jesus humbled himself. He set aside the glory of being God to move into our neighborhood and be one of us. Jesus set aside his glory for you. Don't be fooled into thinking you must accomplish certain standards in order to be worth something. You are made for a relationship with God. Jesus came to show us that relationship.

Don't measure your worth by what you can do or what you look like or what other people think about you. See who you are in God's eyes. Jesus said, "Take my yoke upon you and learn from me, for I am gentle and humble in heart" (Matthew 11:29).

True humility is about being grateful for God's grace in your life and reflecting it in your relationships.

True humility recognizes that everything you have comes from God.

True humility frees you from a pointless search for something to be proud of.

Put on humility toward yourself and take the next step toward wholeness of body-and-spirit. It will be good for your health.

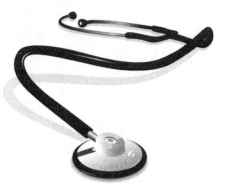

18

Put On Gentleness

More things unite us than divide us.

Mrs. Stephens screeched at me, "My brother told me that you should give me three months' worth of medicine to help me stop smoking. You only gave me enough for one month, so I didn't take it."

I tried to keep my cool. "So where did your brother get this information?"

"He researched thoroughly on the Internet."

This is not my favorite remark to hear, but things got worse. Generally the second time I see a patient, I begin to ask questions about family and social life. She was only fifty years old, so one of my questions was, "What kind of work do you do?"

"What kind of work do I do?" she snapped. "My husband is seventy-three years old. I take care of him."

"Does he have a serious illness?"

"No. He's fine."

At that point I knew Mrs. Stephens lied to us at some point during her initial interview. We would not have given her an appointment if she told us she had no job. While we don't make a value judgment that every person must work, I decided at the beginning of the Church Health Center that our purpose specifically was to care for the working poor who often are in jobs no one else wants to do. While I make exceptions to our guidelines every day, Mrs. Stephens's attitude made it easy to tell her I could not continue to see her unless she decided to seek employment. When I finished my explanation, she screamed at me.

"Where am I supposed to go?"

Calmly I gave her the list of government-funded clinics that would see her and charge her based on her income. Her anger continued unabated.

"I will call every church in this city," she said, "and tell them what this place is really like."

I said nothing more. I left the room and headed to the water fountain, where I drank slowly and tried to decrease my heart rate.

One Friday night a patient called at 9:30, railing about a refill on her diabetes medication. "I saw Dr. Ford two weeks ago and she did not give me enough medicine to last until I come back. I only have one pill left."

We often get calls from people who wait until the last minute to call about their medicine, and it's frustrating. When a patient with a chronic condition has only one pill left, it doesn't leave me a lot of options. I asked, "Why did you wait until the last minute to call? You know the clinic is closed now."

Angry, she replied, "I called three times and no one called me back."

It's not unusual for a patient to tell me this, but I know the clinic nurses often work two hours past the end of their shift in order to return all the calls. This woman insisted no one called her back. I offered to phone in a prescription to the pharmacy of her choice.

"I don't have any money for my prescription," she said, seething. "That's why I come to the Church Health Center."

I knew this was true, but her sense of asserting a right infuriated me. I shot back, "I'm not sure we are going to be able to give you your medicine anymore, but I will be happy to call in a prescription."

"What do you want me to do—die?"

I tried to calm down.

"What is your name?" she demanded.

Her tone told me she planned to report me. I wasn't sure to whom—the radio station talk shows? The mayor? I've been reported to them all in the past. I once again offered to call in a prescription for her immediate need and said she could see Dr. Ford again Monday morning. It was the best I could do at the time.

Gentleness is a choice.

"Therefore as God's chosen people, put on. . .gentleness," Paul wrote to the Colossians. To people living in Philippi he wrote, "Let your gentleness be evident to all" (Philippians 4:5). I suppose if you've put it on and you're wearing it, others will see it. It will be evident. Paul also pleaded with the people in Corinth, "By the meekness and gentleness of Christ. . ." (2 Corinthians 10:1). It would seem people in the first century were just as harsh as the people you and I meet every day.

I don't think Paul was talking about a namby-pamby silly Jesus who let people walk all over him. So why does Paul describe Jesus this way?

Jesus brought us the kingdom of God without using force. He didn't have an army, just a group of friends who too often were thickheaded about what he was doing. Jesus didn't have political clout to swing around. He wasn't a CEO who could snap his fingers and make hundreds of people jump. He didn't pile up money just to prove he could.

Jesus told stories and touched people's faces and answered their questions and healed their broken lives. He brought the kingdom of God and lived its reality in every encounter. That added up to meekness and gentleness. It's not always easy. People push my buttons just the way they push yours.

Gentleness is the image of your mother bending over you and soothing your forehead when things are not going well. It's the image of a mother bird flying down to the chick that fell out of the nest, or that of a mother dog encouraging a puppy. Gentleness may be tender, but it has purpose. Gentleness is a way to approach another human being in a manner that communicates respect and care. It's a consideration for other people that shows up in our willingness to waive our own rights. Our world is so brash. Sometimes the first contact with another person borders on cruelty. We are not willing to give up our rights out of consideration for another person in need, not even our place in line at the grocery store or that parking spot we spied first. We are reluctant even to give up a moment of attention to notice the need of another person.

During medical school, I lived with Howard and Margaret Montgomery. Howard used to be the publisher at John Knox Press. He was a busy and successful man. But when I was with Howard, he was fully present for me. While he was talking to me, he didn't think about a list of other things. He didn't even try to think what he would say next in the conversation. He waived his own rights and was simply and gently there with me.

Tom White was a retired physician who volunteered at the Church Health Center on a full-time basis. He started by agreeing to see patients for twenty hours a week, but within two weeks he asked, "Do you think I could come more often?" The twenty hours expanded to forty, where it stayed for many years.

One busy Monday at the clinic, Tom grabbed my arm. "Do you remember Mrs. Clarke? She's been your patient a long time."

I turned to see Mrs. Clarke, a cheerful woman in her sixties, beaming at me.

"She just got a new kidney," Tom explained.

For twenty years Tom worked as a nephrologist. He was a great resource in helping people with kidney disease, and he orchestrated the surgery in which Mrs. Clarke's youngest son donated a kidney.

I saw the results of Tom's kindness and gentleness with patients most clearly when I treated patients who were used to seeing him. I could sense their disappointment when I walked into the room and I wasn't Tom! One patient said, "No offense, Doc, but Dr. White knows my care good and he is what you call *more mature*." Another said to me, "You look so much younger," and it dawned on me she was used to seeing Tom—who was thirty-five years older than I was—and thought I was him.

When Tom turned eighty, he said, "Scott, you have to promise you'll tell me if I start making mistakes. I couldn't stand to be a burden to this place." He was not about to insist on being the center of attention. He only wanted patients to get the best care we could offer. When he turned eighty-three, Tom decided he no longer would see patients on a daily basis. He continued to review charts, though. When he found errors, he delivered the news with kindness, never pointing the finger of blame. Tom had a gentle way of approaching people in a harsh world that loves to find fault.

Treat yourself with gentleness.

More things unite us than divide us, but we too often focus on what divides. We find fault. We pass the blame. We draw lines and dare someone to step across. We arrange our systems to prove we are right!

Gentleness does just the opposite. Gentleness thinks the best of someone, hopes for the best, encourages the best.

How are you doing at thinking the best of yourself? Perhaps you blame yourself for some difficult situation, and this keeps you from moving through to the healing waiting on the other side. Perhaps you think of yourself in judgmental terms. Perhaps you are the first one in line to criticize yourself.

You know what happens to your sense of well-being when someone else is harsh with you—the defensive instinct, the urge to point fingers back, the drive to take the power in the encounter and come out on top, the increased heart rate, the rattled distraction that follows you for hours or days afterward. The last thing you need is to inflict that on yourself.

As you strive to make healthy choices, to find what brings joy to your life, and to understand that wellness is not just the absence of disease, you'll have some rocky moments. You'll say things you wish you hadn't said and do things you wish you hadn't done. Put on gentleness toward yourself and receive God's grace in those moments. It will be good for your health.

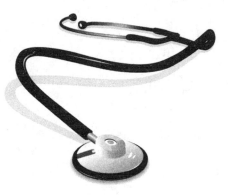

19

Put On Patience

Patience gives God's time a chance to be fulfilled.

The war in Europe was over. Finally back in the States, Clarence and the rest of his unit received the long-awaited news that they were eligible for discharge. Ecstatic, soldiers who came from the same region of Mississippi piled into a bus that would carry them to their assorted small hometowns.

The bus driver sat motionless.

The soldiers settled in, ready to go.

The bus driver did not move.

Finally one of the soldiers asked, "What's wrong? Let's get rolling."

The driver answered, "I ain't driving this bus anywhere until the niggers get in the back."

Clarence's breath caught. He was one of the riders the driver was talking about. He grew up in a tiny Mississippi town where children, black and white, played with each other and scampered from house to house through the front doors. But he was not oblivious to the racism of the South during his childhood.

When his unit briefly was stationed in a small hamlet outside London, soldiers were allowed leave once a week—based on race. The white soldiers went into town on Monday, and the African Americans on Tuesday. "When we got there on Tuesday," Clarence told me years later, "the English girls wanted to know why we weren't there the night before. After we explained how it worked, the next Monday, the girls didn't show up. They waited for us on Tuesday. They said, 'Over here in England there is no discrimination.' "

But this bus driver wasn't in England, and he wanted Clarence at the back of the bus.

The white soldiers were on their feet, incensed and incredulous. "We fought together with these men, we slept in the same holes, and now you're not going to drive the bus because they're sitting with us?"

"Start the bus," someone growled.

When he told me the story, Clarence said, "They roughed him up pretty good and he decided to drive us all home."

Clarence's life was never particularly easy. His father plowed a field in the spring, grew cotton all summer, and ran the local cotton gin in the fall. One day on his way home from school, Clarence found his father throwing up green stuff in the field. His appendix had burst. Because of his father's illness, Clarence dropped out of the sixth grade to follow the mule that heaved the plow through the field to prepare for the crop. It was the only way his family would survive. He never returned to school. A few years later, as a young soldier, Clarence drove an ambulance all over Europe.

After the war, when he moved to Tennessee, Clarence discovered that the experience on the bus would be repeated over and over throughout his life. As he remembered, "I was a country boy, and when I came to the city I found out I couldn't drink out of the same fountains as white folks." But Clarence didn't have any bitter feelings about the unequal treatment he experienced. By the time I met him, he was seventy years old, and I was curious.

"For most of your life," I said, "white people have treated you unjustly. They've abused you in various ways and seen you as less than a man. Yet you have not allowed yourself to become bitter."

That's when Clarence told me the story of the bus. He was one person, and his anger around racism probably was not going to change the world. But in that moment on the bus, he saw the fruit of patience. Before the war, these white soldiers likely would not have given Clarence the time of day. Now they adamantly rose to his defense. Now they saw him for who he was, not as something less than human. He was an equal who not only had a right to sit where he wanted to on the bus, but whose blood was just as red as theirs and who loved his family as much as they did. He had desires and aspirations and hopes for a better life just as they did. He could have told them all this much earlier, if they had cared, but now they knew it for themselves. Clarence hadn't changed; they had.

Clarence would say that this change came about because of his patience. From that point on, and for fifty years until the day I met him, he remembered that experience. It became his model for how he approached similar situations. Ultimately, Clarence believed God was in control even of experiences of injustice. On the bus that day, Clarence glimpsed God's mercy coming to fullness in his life—what it could be and will be someday in the kingdom of God. He continued to bump up against racism in the decades that followed, but he never let anger control him. Instead, he lived his life with his eyes on what it meant to be a disciple of Jesus, including patient expectation that God could change people. Living with patience gave him peace and tranquility in his life, even when others wondered how he could endure what happened to him. In spite of injustice, Clarence was happy.

We wait for God.

Who doesn't want to be more patient? Probably, though, you don't need all the fingers on one hand to name the people you know who truly are patient. Even people you consider patient can tell you a million ways they're not. Do people really want patience, or is it a fantasy?

Most of us are content with impatience, or even see patience as a weakness. Waiting too long for a table at a restaurant is foolish. Waiting more than ninety seconds at the grocery checkout is a cosmic injustice. Going at the pace of a child is akin to taking a stroll with a slug. If a Web site requires more than two seconds to appear on your computer screen, it doesn't deserve your attention. One of the most common appeals for sympathy is "I had to wait," as if we can think of nothing worse.

Most of our impatience has to do with not getting what we want fast enough. We want it, and we want it now. On a surface level, being patient amounts to a willingness to wait longer than you should have to. And the cultural message is that if you're patient, someone is likely to take advantage of you. Standing up for yourself—demanding your "right" to faster food or whatever—is a higher cultural value than being patient and possibly losing out. That's what our culture says.

But what if that is not the essence of patience?

What if patience means putting up with the sometimes exasperating choices of others, even enduring wrong, because you are waiting for God to bring about change? The New Testament book of James has a great section on patience:

> Brothers, as an example of patience in the face of suffering,
> take the prophets who spoke in the name of the Lord. As
> you know, we consider blessed those who have persevered.
> You have heard of Job's perseverance and have seen what the

Lord finally brought about. The Lord is full of compassion and mercy. (James 5:10–11)

Elijah spoke the word of God and had to run for his life from Jezebel, a crazed queen with a penchant for slaughtering prophets. Jeremiah was thrown into a muddy cistern as a reward for his hard work speaking God's messages to people who could not have cared less. Being a prophet in Old Testament times was not a cushy job. Prophets had to have the long term in mind, not immediate gratification. They were part of what God was doing and waited for God's movement, in God's time. We refer to the "patience of Job" because he endured so much suffering, yet refused to believe God had abandoned him. "I know that my Redeemer lives," Job said, "and that in the end he will stand upon the earth" (Job 19:25).

With these examples, James reminds us of "what the Lord finally brought about" because God is by nature full of compassion and mercy. Patience is about waiting on God. We wait not for God to do what we think God should do, but for the fullness of God to be revealed. We wait—expectantly—for God's Spirit to manifest in our circumstances and relationships. This does not always happen as quickly as we might like or in the way we might hope. Patience is a bit like putting pennies in a piggy bank to save for something you want. Adding just a little at a time, it might seem that the bank will never be full enough—until it is.

When the time comes, God moves. That's the lesson Clarence learned on the bus. The point of patience is not to wait without complaining for what we want to get, but to wait expectantly for what God wants to give. Through patience in relationships, we share God's grace with each other. Through patience in suffering, we open ourselves to new ways of experiencing God's presence. Patience gives God's time a chance to be fulfilled.

Treat yourself with patience.

Wellness does not happen overnight. Even if you decide to take the turn toward wellness, the road still stretches before you. The potholes are still there and you may well fall into them again. You may need to form some new habits when it comes to the food you eat, your activity level, the nature of your relationships, and attitudes toward your work. This takes time. A "hurry and get healthy" approach seldom leads to better long-term health. Be patient with the time it takes, and remember that God does not say, "This is what wholeness looks like, so go do it." God is with you on the journey. We are whole body-and-spirit beings created and loved by God.

Avoid the pothole of thinking that if you have to wait for results, the effort is lacking. Losing weight takes time. Sorting out relationships takes time. Discovering what fills you with joy takes time. Accomplishing goals happens one step at a time, not in a moment of instant gratification.

Rejoice in what God brings about in your life because of compassion and mercy. Treat yourself with patience. It will be good for your health.

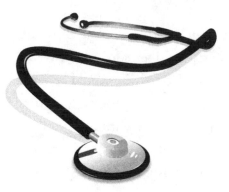

20

Put On Forgiveness

We are going to disappoint each other.

Erma's youthful marriage was impetuous and short-lived. When she and her husband parted ways, she became a single mother with two small children. For the next fifteen years, Erma moved from one clerical job to the next, trying to earn more money. Then when her son was seventeen, the landscape shifted violently.

On a summer Tuesday, Erma's son, Milton, left home at about seven in the evening. He was headed to a shoe store that was open until nine, so he had plenty of time to make the trip on the bus. Tall and lanky, Milton towered above the others waiting on the corner for the bus. Just down the block, a group of teenage boys loitered. Suddenly another boy ran up to the group, elated. He had just stolen a gun from his brother-in-law and was eager to show off his loot. The gun ignited teenage energy and they couldn't pass it around fast enough. Somehow the trigger was pulled while the gun was haphazardly pointed toward the bus stop.

The bullet hit Milton in the head. He died instantly.

Erma didn't want to believe what everyone was saying when they arrived at her door. Her son was just going on an ordinary errand to the shoe store. Surely he would be home soon. She waited for his knock at the door, and it took a long time for the feeling to fade that he would be home any minute.

The one person missing from Milton's funeral was the boy who pulled the trigger. He was a friend of Milton's, but how could he face Erma now?

"I pondered what to believe and I knew I had to pray," Erma told me twenty-three years later. "What if that were my son? I would want someone to show mercy." Erma lost her son, but she never felt bitterness toward the boy who caused her loss. "He was punished enough," she said.

Erma went to see the boy who had been too ashamed to come to the funeral. "I love you," she told him. "I don't believe you deliberately shot my son."

Some of Erma's church friends doubted her love for her son at that time. "They felt like I didn't have the grief I should have," she told me, "but God promised to be with me always. The Spirit spoke to me. God doesn't make mistakes. God gave me consolation. I didn't make it hard for his family. I could only show love."

Erma was telling me her life story because she had a question. Her now-grown daughter had a son serving a term in prison, while his former teenage girlfriend was losing interest in their child. Erma planned to drive to Illinois and bring back her great-granddaughter. She told me, "I want her to grow up knowing she is loved." Erma wanted me to be the girl's doctor. Of course I said yes, if for no other reason than the chance to be with a person who took seriously the call to forgive those who wrong us. If I lived the trauma Erma endured, the lure of bitterness would be strong. But Erma found a way to turn the greatest evil in her life into a source from which love springs daily.

Forgiveness heals.

Even in her loss, Erma put herself in someone else's shoes, and it made all the difference. "What if it were my son?"

This certainly was not Peter's instinct. In Matthew 18, we read how Jesus was teaching about how to handle situations when one person wrongs another. It's going to happen. That's why Jesus talked about restoration of relationships in the first place. Against this backdrop, Peter, one of Jesus' inner circle of friends, asked essentially, "When is enough, enough? How serious is this business about forgiveness?" When Peter offered to forgive a repeat offender seven times, he no doubt thought he was being quite generous. Imagine Peter's shock when Jesus answered, "Buzz! Wrong answer! Stop putting boundaries around forgiveness."

Jesus then told a story of two servants. One owed the king millions of dollars, far beyond his ability to ever settle the debt. When he threw himself on the king's mercy, the king compassionately canceled the debt. Exuberant, the servant went on his merry way. When he crossed paths with another servant who owed him a few pennies by comparison, he demanded repayment of the loan immediately. Though the debt was small, the second man could not repay it any more than the first could repay his enormous debt. But rather than learning from his experience of mercy and putting himself in the shoes of his fellow worker, the first servant had the second one thrown into debtor's prison, which technically he had the right to do. When the king got wind of this, he was less than pleased. "Shouldn't you have had mercy on your fellow servant," he asked, "just as I had on you?" (Matthew 18:33).

"Bear with each other," Paul says in the Colossians 3 virtues passage, "and forgive whatever grievances you may have against one another. Forgive as the Lord forgave you."

Paul knows relationships are going to hit snags. We're going to annoy each other. We're going to disappoint each other. We're going to wound each other. Deeply. We're going to think there's no going back. Being clothed with compassion, kindness, humility, gentleness, and patience gives way to being able to bear with each other in these moments. By God's grace we glimpse a reality bigger than the offense that causes our pain. Bearing with each other, and the forgiveness that results, has nothing to do with deserving it. Paul loves to remind readers of God's unconditional love for them and God's unbounded forgiveness. This is the basis of our forgiveness of one another. We forgive because we have been forgiven. We offer gracious pardon to those who offend us because we know God's gracious pardon of us.

Forgiveness is healing to the one who is forgiven. This we experience most fully in God's forgiveness of us. God's forgiveness of our offenses restores our relationship with God, and we have a picture of the healing we can offer to others in forgiveness. This gift keeps us in community with people who care for us by building bridges rather than tearing them down and walking away.

Forgiveness also is healing to the person who forgives. This we experience when we forgive others. When we offer forgiveness, we receive the healing that comes from letting go of the grievance and being no longer held captive by a thirst for vengeance. This means less anxiety and depression and a better overall sense of well-being. It means having more energy to devote to what brings joy rather than wasting energy on what does not.

Treat yourself with forgiveness.

We all make mistakes. Sometimes—perhaps most of the time—we argue our way out of thinking we did anything wrong. We scrounge up all sorts of reasons to justify a sharp word or harsh action that harms someone else. Our excuses point fingers at another person or circumstance beyond our control. It's not our fault.

Sometimes, though, we do own up. We've done wrong, and

we know it. Now it's time to make things right. Forgiving another person is good for your health. Do you owe someone an apology? Have you hurt someone, whether you meant to or not? Are you harboring an offense even if outwardly you say it doesn't matter? Perhaps it is time to let go of being right so you can experience joy in that relationship. By offering forgiveness and restoring the relationship, you can bring healing both to yourself and to the other person. Follow Erma's example and put yourself in someone else's shoes.

And what anger are you holding against yourself? Perhaps you just cannot get past a decision or impulsive act that brought harmful or lasting consequences to your life. Maybe you're stuck in a habit you despise but can't seem to quit. Perhaps hateful words ring in your head because you can't believe they came out of your mouth. Maybe you've fallen far short of your expectations for yourself. It's time to forgive yourself, just as God has forgiven you.

The point of forgiveness is restoration and a return to wholeness of relationship. That includes the health of your relationship with yourself. How you see yourself colors how you see other people. You don't have to be stuck for the rest of your life with a picture of yourself that says you deserve your misery when God has arms open wide to forgive you.

Treat yourself with forgiveness. It will be good for your health.

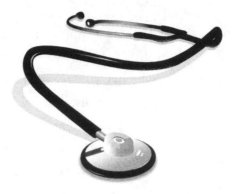

21

Put On Love, the Binding Agent

This love does not come from Hollywood.

Margaret was in her midfifties when an aneurysm ruptured in her brain and produced a stroke. She recovered most of her physical function, but her mental function was never quite the same. For one thing, she couldn't seem to control the connection between her thoughts and her tongue. If she thought it, she said it, whether it was appropriate or not. At the same time, though, she struggled for words. Her husband of thirty years functioned as her interpreter, but Margaret got frustrated when she couldn't form her thoughts appropriately or if Henry didn't understand her. Her frustration relief valve, unfortunately, was to cuss at Henry and kick him in the shins until he figured out what she wanted him to say. Henry accepted whatever Margaret dished out. Whenever I saw them, I was touched by Henry's devotion to Margaret and what he put up with. It was clear to me that Margaret always thought she would eventually get better, but medically that seemed unlikely considering the amount of time that had passed since the stroke.

One day the two of them came to see me for a regular visit,

but they were not their regular selves. Henry, especially, seemed off. Finally he told me that their daughter had committed suicide by taking an overdose of Tylenol, which is an incredibly slow and painful way to die. Even after reaching a point of no return in the physical effect of the drug, it takes days to die of this kind of overdose. Their daughter was taken to a hospital and admitted to the intensive care unit, but it was inevitable she was going to die.

Just before she slipped into a coma, she looked up and said, "Daddy, can you ever forgive me?"

Henry answered, "You know that your mother and I have always loved you and always will."

As Henry told me this story, Margaret reached for his hand and gripped it. She understood Henry's love for her as well, even though she would never get any better medically than she was.

A few years ago I had joint replacement surgery, which is no picnic. When you go through something like that, you need somebody with you. I experienced incredible incapacitation and loss of autonomy, just like anyone else who has a knee or hip replaced. Suddenly every basic daily need requires assistance. At no turn did my wife, Mary, ever turn away. She's not a nurse; she's an actress, but she rolled up her sleeves and did whatever it took. While I still struggled mightily in the hospital, Mary announced we were going home. I protested and pleaded that I was not ready, but she got me in a wheelchair and made me get in the car and took me home, up the stairs, and to my own bed and my Bernese mountain dogs. I hope that if my wife ever needs me to do that for her, I would be able to reciprocate.

Thelma was in her sixties and earning minimum wage working at a laundry facility. She had been paying on her small house for over twenty years and just about had it paid off. Her son recently had married and celebrated a new baby. Thelma planned to give her house to her son. "It's only me in the house," she told me, "and he needs a place where he can raise his family. God only gives to us so we can give to others."

"Where will you live?" I asked.

"I'll find somewhere. I don't need much."

There's nothing glamorous about this kind of sacrificial love. You do what needs to be done because you have a passion for another person, but not in the way we typically understand passion. This kind of passion is devoted to seeing that person made whole, no matter what the circumstance.

Love is the final garment.

People have a vision of love shaped by Hollywood and those first pangs of the teenage heart. The American myth of the lonesome cowboy—Clint Eastwood in spaghetti westerns—may be romantic for two hours, but no one should attempt that at home. That's not life as it's meant to be lived. Real love—a passion for the wholeness of another person—does not mean everything is sweetness and light. Being healthy does not mean you don't face challenges. But love provides the strength to deal with the adversity of life. This love does not come from Hollywood.

As we put on the new clothes God gives us, the final garment is love. Paul says, "And over all these virtues put on love, which binds them all together in perfect unity" (Colossians 3:14). This abiding underlying principle holds all the virtues in place. Without love, the rest of the ensemble goes askew.

Jesus knew God loved him. He knew the power of love. Moments before he was arrested and began his walk to the cross, Jesus prayed for all who would believe in him. The final words of his prayer were:

Father, I want those you have given me to be with me where I am, and to see my glory, the glory you have given me because you loved me before the creation of the world. . . .

I have made you known to them, and will continue to make
you known in order that the love you have for me may be in
them and that I myself may be in them. (John 17:24, 26)

Love doesn't come from Hollywood. It comes from God. God
loved Jesus, and Jesus revealed God to us. Out of love, God sent
Jesus. Out of love, Jesus sacrificed himself so that we could be
connected to God without any barrier in between. And out of our
experience of God's love, we love others. Paul wrote to the Romans
that all God's commandments are summed up in the simple phrase,
"Love your neighbor as yourself" (Romans 13:9).

God's love is not mere sentimental feeling. It's not an impulse.
It's not rooted in an irresistible "chemistry." When we look at what
God did through Jesus, we see motive and intention. We see choice
and action. We see pain and sacrifice. This love is not about feeling
good, as if life were a romantic comedy. Rather, love is a profound
dedication and sense of commitment to another human being.
It might actually be painful at times, but powerful motive and
deliberate choice come to the forefront because love has its eye on
the well-being of another person. Love will do what it takes to help
that person experience more wholeness—health—as a body-and-
spirit being created and loved by God. Love lets people continue
to move forward despite the pain and suffering life can bring. Love
enables people to believe life is good and meaningful when you
might otherwise wring your hands and say, "Why me, Lord?"

The other virtues—compassion, kindness, humility, gentleness,
patience, forgiveness—make sense because love is the engine of life.
It's the essence of who we are as human beings. If the other virtues
are characteristics of God, love is the unsurpassed demonstration of
how God wants to relate to us, and how God wants us to relate to
each other. Love binds the other virtues together in maturity and
fullness—perfect unity.

Treat yourself with love.

If you believe God loves everyone with a powerful motive and deliberate choice, do you also believe God loves you? Human beings have a pervasive capacity to doubt. We can actually agree, on one hand, that God is love and loves all people, and believer, on the other hand, that God does not love me.

We tell ourselves, "If God really loved me, my life would not be so hard." But God loved Jesus, and Jesus suffered an excruciating death he did not deserve.

We convince ourselves, "Even God could not love me after what I've done." We miss the truth that God does not love us because we deserve it, but because God chooses to.

We look through the mirror the wrong way and measure God's love according to how it reflects our experience of failed human love. Instead, we need to see that love begins in the heart of God and we reflect it in our relationships.

God loves you.

The next person who needs to love you is *you*. Paul did not say, "Love yourself the way you love your neighbor." He said, "Love your neighbor as you love yourself." Before Paul, Jesus said this, and centuries before Jesus' earthly ministry, God said this to Moses and the ancient Israelites. Loving yourself is fundamental to your health. It's essential to caring for yourself.

Do you somehow think God doesn't love you, not really?

Do you feel there is nothing lovable in you?

Are you so stressed by the demands of your life that treating yourself with love doesn't even make the list of what you will attempt?

Treat yourself with love. It will be good for your health.

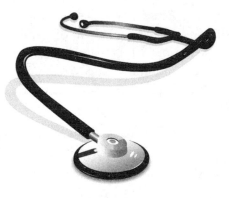

22

You Decide Your Own Health Care

You are the expert in your own health care.

There's a reason why a company will offer a million dollars to a fan who can kick a field goal during halftime at the Super Bowl. It's a safe bet that the selected fan has not practiced enough nor developed enough skill to succeed. Everyone hopes the kicker will win the million dollars, and there's always a random chance. Wouldn't it be cool if the random chance happened before our eyes? On national television with millions of people watching? It could happen. People play the lottery for the same reason—even if the odds are 38 billion to 1, there's always a random chance, and wouldn't it be incredible if that random winner was you? We waste massive amounts of money hoping for that random chance. When someone does win the lottery, or suddenly becomes wealthy for any reason, the inevitable question is, "How will this change your life?"

The beauty of life is that you don't have to win the lottery for life to be wonderful. God's plan for us is about enjoying life day in and day out, not just at the extremes where we hope something miraculous will happen. Life can be full of wonder every day if we choose it.

Practice matters.

Far too many people expect something that is unlikely to happen simply by random chance. More often than we think, though, we can make choices that bring the "wow" factor to our lives in a more realistic way. Part of being healthy and living a whole life is avoiding those moments when we feel like we're cramming for a final exam and everything depends on the outcome of this one test. Every class has the student who perpetually asks, "Is it going to be on the test?" Teachers sigh and try another angle to interest students in real learning that lasts a lifetime, not just long enough for the exam. Always doing the minimum to catch up to where you should have been last week is no way to live. It's not healthy. It doesn't make you well. It doesn't allow you to feel whole, even if you do kick an astounding field goal once in a while.

Practice matters. If you exercise on a regular basis, for instance, your body will deal better with an injury or unexpected physical demands beyond your usual life. If you eat well, your body will have richer resources to draw on at times of pressure or healing. If you have a pattern for how you relate to God, that pattern will kick in and sustain you in times of tension and questioning. The professional basketball player who makes the game-winning, three-point shot just before the clock buzzes doesn't do it because of a random moment. He does it because he has shot thousands of practice shots. Some he made; some he missed. But he did it over and over and learned something every time. When millions of people are watching and the game is on the line, muscle memory kicks in and he makes the shot.

Living a healthy life is a lot like that. Without practice, few play the game well under stress. Without practiced patterns, we lack a meaningful context for important decisions. Without practiced patterns, sudden stress knocks us off our feet. Without practiced patterns, we are clueless about end-of-life decisions involving ourselves or our loved ones. Without practiced patterns, illness is stronger than we are. Without practiced patterns, suffering throws us into a tailspin.

Decision moments come at unexpected times. If you have not examined what's important to you in times of calm, you won't know how to respond in times of stress. It's horrendously challenging to make sound decisions under pressure. For instance, if a loved one has an accident and is suddenly on life support, and the doctor asks you what to do, will you know? If you haven't had that conversation at a time of calm and wellness, you'll be stymied in a time of turmoil. If the bottom falls out of your finances because of something you never saw coming, will you respond out of panic or out of knowing what's important to you? If a relationship disintegrates before your eyes, will you feel abandoned and bereft, or will you know you are a precious human being? If disease strikes and you have to make decisions about treatment and recovery, will you have a base of values to guide you? Without practice at living life well, we might just as well flip a coin in these situations.

You can develop a way of living that gives you joy akin to winning the lottery. You can take steps toward health care you can live with.

Know yourself.

We see so many people at the Church Health Center and our Wellness facility who are isolated. Not only are they isolated from other people and lack nurturing and sustaining relationships, but they are isolated from themselves. They may come to us with illnesses or physical conditions, but the more substantial question is this: What causes the behaviors that lead to the physical distress? So often patients don't make the connection. They may understand, for instance, that eating too much causes them to carry an unhealthy weight. But why do they eat the way they do? That they may not know. They haven't connected the dots between the stress factors in their lives and their eating habits. And it's unlikely their eating habits will change until they do connect the dots. It's difficult to change behaviors if the core reason behind the behavior doesn't change.

This is why we stress the virtues of Colossians 3 in our health care ministry. Absorbing the virtues and demonstrating them toward others and ourselves is the beginning of changing the core issues that drive unhealthy behaviors. Unhealthy behaviors result in a range of common diseases, from obesity to diabetes, from alcoholism to substance abuse, from high blood pressure to high cholesterol and related heart disease. All of these common conditions tax the health care system, but ultimately technology is not the answer. Most of the time they can be prevented or well managed and do not have to become crises.

It comes down to personal choice to change, and change starts in identifying what's wrong in the first place. If eating in unhealthy ways is a response to stress, then what can you do to change or manage the source of pressure by seeing the virtues at work in your life? If a sedentary lifestyle is a depressed response to hating your job, then what can you do to change your job, or change how you respond to it with the virtues? If you'd rather play video games alone because you're sure no one wants to be your friend anyway, what is it that makes you feel so worthless?

What is the question behind the question? Real change in health begins here, not in hospital technology. This is the place where experiencing the virtues can make a difference. If the virtues are not a part of your life, guiding your choices, values, and relationships, then making choices that lead to a fuller, more whole life won't matter to you. If you don't feel good about your ability to be a whole person for yourself and others, you will have a terrible time navigating the kinds of change that will make you healthier physically and spiritually.

Change happens over time, not overnight.

Being healthy doesn't happen because one day you wake up and decide to be healthy. Deciding you want to be a size six is not going to make you a size six. Deciding you don't want to have high blood pressure is not going to abolish your hypertension. This is a common pitfall. People believe that overnight they can just stop doing the things that bog them down. In reality, movement toward health is a process of change, a series of choices—and it happens over time, not overnight.

Burt was one of the first members of Church Health Center Wellness when it opened. He weighed over five hundred pounds. One day after he had been coming to Wellness regularly for about a year, he walked in and said, "You won't believe this, but I got my car back!"

"That's great!" We had no idea he had lost his car.

Burt was so morbidly obese that he couldn't get behind the steering wheel of a car. After a year, he had lost enough weight to get in his car. Was he still morbidly overweight? Yes. But he was moving toward health, and he was closer to a healthy weight than he had been a year before.

A woman came in one day and told us that for the first time in ten years, she could make her bed without stopping in the middle of the task to catch her breath. Whether you have to rest in the middle of making your bed doesn't show up in any statistical measurements of health, but for her it was a huge indicator of movement toward health.

Foundations and researchers tend to want to quantify everything. They'll tell you how much you *should* weigh, how much exercise you *should* get, how many calories you *should* consume.

They'll tell you whether this weight loss plan or that exercise program statistically resulted in better health in the groups they studied. Generally, though, they don't measure the impact of faith and community on health. People who can't get behind the wheel of a car or make their beds without losing their breath are so far outside the boundaries of "healthy" that researchers hardly know what to do with them. Yet these two people who used our Wellness facility—with the support of faith and community—clearly moved to a better level of health.

You might be a 2 on a scale of 1 to 10. You're not going to be a 10 in the morning or by a week from Monday. You're not even going to be an 8 or a 6. But perhaps you will move to a 3 by the next time you see your doctor.

You're in charge.

You are the expert in your own health care, and you can be in charge of this process. Perhaps you are coming out of years of being unaware or unconvinced of the need for change, and now you're thinking about it. Perhaps you even intend to change, and the virtues of Colossians 3 will sustain you through the process. Next comes action. Next comes your future.

Most people—not all—in their twenties are free of major disease by virtue of their youth. Even in their thirties, people who have an annual physical are unlikely to come away with any news. The chance that a doctor will find something in a person with no symptoms is close to zero. What does make sense for the annual physical, though, is to look at where you are on the spectrum of wellness. Where are you in experiencing the virtues? Where are you in understanding the causes of some of your behaviors? Where are you in finding joy in your life? How do the answers to these questions affect your body? Are you moving from a 2 to a 3 to a 5? Individual choices to practice healthy behaviors come down to caring for the body God gave us because we understand we are whole beings created and loved by God, body-and-spirit.

Understanding yourself and making choices apart from a crisis can prevent disease later. Prevention looks at the big picture over a period of time, not at immediate gratification. Exploring the whole meaning of wellness for body-and-spirit allows you to decide on your own health care because you are actively caring for the whole you, rather than waiting for a doctor to fix you after you break. You *can* take the turn and decide to practice good health behaviors and truly love the body God gave you.

Choose the wonder of life. It will be good for your health.

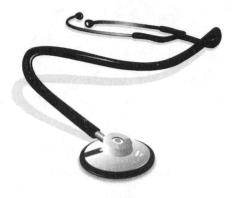

23

Discover the Balance

Small things make life better.

So how do we turn the virtues of Colossians 3 into a plan for healthier living? We've wrestled with this question at the Church Health Center. It's why our Wellness facility exists. Reminders of virtues are everywhere in the building, and we talk about them a lot. But how do they lead to change? Over the years we've recognized the need for each person to have an individual plan for wellness. We developed the Model for Healthy Living as a tool to help people choose ways to care for their own health.

We don't start with the doctor; we start with the health coach.

When new patients—without an urgent illness—come to the Church Health Center, their first stop is our Wellness facility. They may simply be getting established with a new doctor for future care, or they may have conditions that need to be monitored, though they are not sick at the time. The first conversation with a health coach introduces the concept of overall wellness, not simply medical issues. Patients fill out a questionnaire that covers the usual health history, but also ventures into questions that give us clues about the patient's life beyond chronic conditions or what might be hurting at the moment. Here are a few of our questions:

"Are you satisfied with your spiritual life?"

"How strongly religious (or spiritually oriented) do you consider yourself to be?"

"Which of the following would you most prefer from your health care team? Never ask you about your spiritual or religious beliefs. Sometimes ask you about your beliefs depending on the situation. Always know about your beliefs."

"In an average week, how often do you eat at least five servings of fruit and vegetables each day?"

"Which answer best describes how you feel about making changes to your eating habits?"

"How often do you experience levels of stress and/or anxiety that affect your ability to function each day?"

"Are you taking care of someone who is elderly, sick, or disabled?"

"How often do you run out of food?"

"In the last year, how often have you needed help to pay your rent, mortgage, and/or utilities?"

Simply scanning the answers to these questions gives the health coach an idea of how open the patient is to talking about faith and how ready the patient might be to make changes—even small ones—to improve overall wellness. This conversation does not say, "Tell me where your body hurts," but rather "Tell me about your life." The health coach helps identify areas where the patient seems to be doing well, along with areas of everyday life that may be negatively affecting health. This session lasts about thirty minutes, and for the most part, people open up. They appreciate the opportunity to talk about their lives with someone who cares.

Sharon met a new patient who was agitated because she had not seen a doctor in years and was worried about the damage she may have done to her body over time. She shared with Sharon that she was gay and that she'd struggled with crack addiction in the past, including being sober for five years, relapsing for three, and now sober again for a year. She was doing this all on her own—no twelve-step program or counseling. They talked about her relationships, her ability to deal with addiction, her support systems, and her work environment. She had few friends and was cut off from her family. Sharon offered some help with developing coping skills and creating a support system, beginning with a referral for counseling. They decided to meet again after the woman saw a counselor. All this happened before the patient met a nurse or a doctor.

Some take longer than others to realize the invitation to talk is sincere, and that's part of the point of allowing a full thirty minutes. It might take twenty-five minutes for a patient to grasp that change is possible, even in small steps. Because it happens in the Wellness center, the session also introduces the patient to services we offer that they might not otherwise be aware of.

After this thirty-minute session, the nurse enters the process in the way you would expect in most clinics, and then the doctor. Future appointments with doctors take place in our main clinic, but now the patient knows Wellness exists. Not everyone returns to Wellness, of course. The idea of self-care is new to a lot of people. Whether or not the patient returns, we have planted the seed for an understanding of healthy living.

One woman was a regular in cooking classes, the pool, and exercise classes for a couple of years. She joined a weight-loss support group, lost some weight, and was doing well. Then she seemed to disappear. After a while, her health coach telephoned her and she admitted she was struggling with some issues. She promised to come back. When she rejoined the exercise class, though, she didn't seem to be herself, so the coach sought her out for a private conversation. She shared that her doctor had sent her for a gastric bypass evaluation and she failed the psychological portion. Now she was distraught, desperate to lose weight so she could have the knee surgery she needed to relieve pain.

After a couple of coaching sessions, the coach believed the woman was a victim of spousal abuse and didn't know it. She failed the psychological evaluation because she didn't have a support system in place for care after surgery. Slowly the truth dawned on the woman that verbal abuse was a form of battering, and she had lived with it for years. The health coach was able to help the woman see how this had affected her health and wellness for a long time.

All the parts connect at the core.

Life is a complicated web, interconnected at every turn. The various parts of our lives bump up against each other. When a relationship is out of whack, you may feel out of whack spiritually as well, or have less enthusiasm for your work. If you hate your job, you may snap at your kids. If you run on fast food and eat on the go, you won't be much interested in exercise. If you sit all day at work, then come home and sit in front of the television, it won't be a surprise that you lie in bed awake at night.

We plan ways to help people understand and incorporate the virtues into their lives. The virtues are in the artwork, even the floor tiles. Ever-present images of the virtues remind people that we don't expect them to make choices to move toward wholeness without the support of the community around them. And we don't expect drastic change all at once. The virtues help people see that change is a process that brings results in the long term.

The virtues are marching orders for how to live. They are overarching ideals that we must translate into specific actions— how to accomplish change. And in that context, we introduce our Model for Healthy Living. This model is a tool for individuals to use to take charge of their own health care, and it reflects that true wellness is not just about our bodies, but about body-and-spirit. We illustrate visually how seven key dimensions of our body-and-spirit experience overlap at the core of our lives.

Nutrition. Good nutrition builds strong bodies that can lead to being whole people better connected to God. What you eat matters. Whatever your eating habits are now, you *can* increase your understanding of how food affects your overall well-being, learn to make smart food choices, and develop healthy eating habits.

Friends and Family. God, Jesus, and the Holy Spirit were the very first relationship. Even God exists in community. Coping with life is sometimes hard, but friends and family make it easier. You *can* both give and receive support through the relationships in your life.

Emotional Life. It's pretty easy to turn to unhealthy habits in response to stress in our lives. For many people, that habit— whether food, mindless television viewing, excessive spending, alcohol, or something else—makes us momentarily feel better even though we know it's bad in the long term. Through understanding your feelings and emotional needs, you *can* make changes to take better care of yourself and manage stress in healthier ways.

Work. We were made to work, and the value of work is intrinsic. You *can* appreciate the skills, talents, and gifts you bring to your work situation, whatever it is. You can find meaning for your life through your job or volunteer commitments.

Movement. We were created to move. When you consider the way the parts of the body are hinged together and rotate and reach in every direction, it's easy to see that God means for us to move. It's part of how we celebrate our body-and-spirit connection to God. No matter what your physical activity level is now, you *can* discover ways to enjoy movement.

Medical Care. You are the expert in your own health care. Your doctor is your partner. Yes, doctors have education, training, and experience you don't have, but you know yourself better than any doctor ever will. When it comes to your medical care, you bring something important to the conversation. You *can* build a partnership with your health care provider that lets you participate in managing your medical care.

Faith Life. We have moved a universe away from seeing faith as an important part of health, and it's time to bring the two back together. Faith traditions vary widely, but at the core, a faith life helps us build a relationship with God, our neighbors, and ourselves. This affirms that we are body-and-spirit beings created and loved by God. Even if you don't consider yourself "religious," you *can* explore a richer faith life and enjoy the benefits this experience will bring to your overall wellness.

In the chapters that follow, we'll look at each of these dimensions more closely, and you'll have an opportunity to identify your own strengths and set personal goals for your own health.

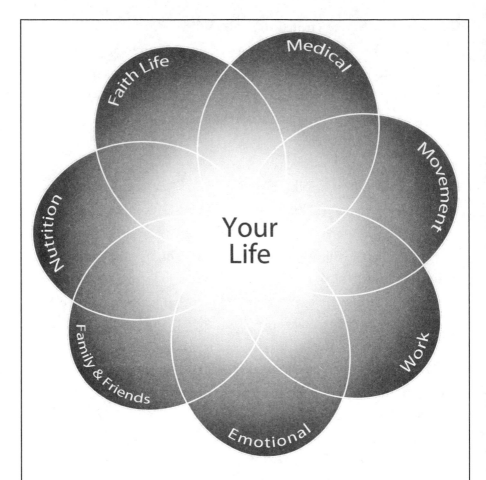

MODEL FOR HEALTHY LIVING

NUTRITION: making smart food choices and eating habits

FRIENDS AND FAMILY: giving and receiving support through relationships

EMOTIONAL LIFE: managing stress and understanding feelings to better care for yourself

WORK: appreciating your skills, talents, and gifts

MOVEMENT: discovering ways to enjoy physical activity

MEDICAL CARE: partnering with health care provider to manage medical care

FAITH LIFE: building a relationship with God, neighbors, and self

Where is your balance point for wellness?

Growing up in Atlanta, I looked forward every year at Christmastime to going to Rich's, a large department store downtown. When I was small, I would go to see Santa, but the main attraction was a train that the store erected in the toy department. Painted like a pink pig, the train ran along the ceiling, and from that viewpoint, kids could see everything the store had to offer. Kids would wait in line forever to ride the pink pig, and when they got off, they received a sticker that said, I RODE THE PINK PIG AT RICH'S. I would wear that sticker from Thanksgiving to Christmas and drive my mother crazy. The last time I rode the pink pig, I was sixteen years old. Many people would have said I was far too old, but I didn't care. I put the sticker on my steering wheel and left it there until I got rid of that car.

We all have these symbols of comfort in our lives. They're different for everyone, and we can't predict what will bring comfort to another person. They give us a sense that all is right with the world after all, and that sense is important to living a healthy life. Nobody should abruptly try to pull away these signs of comfort from another person. You're ready when you're ready. But change does come. I did stop riding the pink pig, as much as I loved it, and you *can* decide that it's time to let go of a habit or way of relating that is no longer healthy for you. At the same time, though, you may develop some new signs of comfort and enjoy sharing them with the people in your life on your journey to wellness. Be open to other people's quirks and not just your own. Be able to laugh. Tell stories like the pink pig. Small things make life better.

It's all about balance. No one of the seven elements in the Model for Healthy Living is more important than any of the others. Each has critical weight in your life and overall wellness. If you ignore one, the whole model goes out of balance. If you overemphasize one, the whole model goes out of balance. If you touch one part of a mobile, the whole mobile moves, responds, and readjusts.

The balance is not the same for everyone. We're not trying to create Stepford wives. Rather, we are trying to help people live faithful lives that allow them to be connected to God. These seven elements are present in every person living in a healthy way, body-and-spirit.

The Model for Healthy Living gives you some framework for change. Specific goals in these seven areas will get you where you want to go. We'll take a look at how to make effective goals, then look more closely at each of the seven dimensions of the Model for Healthy Living.

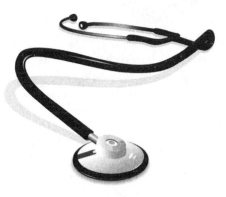

24

Make Goals You Can Keep

Meet yourself where you are.

Taking charge of your health care is a dynamic experience. The right combination of energy and force must come together to produce a particular action or result. The starting point is understanding that you are a body-and-spirit being created and loved by God. When you grasp this, you glimpse the level of health—wholeness, well-being, connection to God and others—that God means for you to experience. As you take the turn toward wholeness, the virtues of Colossians 3 surround you: compassion, kindness, humility, gentleness, patience, forgiveness, and love. You receive these graces from God and more and more learn to give them to others and yourself. This is the context where change can succeed.

In the early stages of change, you want to be sure that what you expect to gain will outweigh what you give up. Will cutting back on comfort foods really make enough difference in my health to be worth the sacrifice? Will joining a support group really make it easier to go through a tough time? Will finding more time to enjoy friends and family really make me happier at work? Will exercise really improve my sleep? If you become convinced that the benefits of change outweigh the demands, you're ready to take steps to change. But *convinced* and *confident* are two different things. You can be convinced of the benefits of change without being confident you can succeed at shifting your own behaviors.

Goals are indispensable to changing behaviors and moving along the wellness spectrum. But a weak goal can do more damage than good, making you feel as if you are moving backward rather than forward. From there it's a short step to deciding it's not worth it to keep trying. On the other hand, strong goals bring focus to succeeding with change.

To begin with, meet yourself where you are. Trying to be something you are not consumes valuable energy—energy you could be putting into healthy choices. Find your genuine starting point, not one you think is more socially acceptable. If you don't eat any vegetables, don't pretend you do. If you work too much, admit it. If you skip church most of the time, don't say you go regularly. Tell yourself the truth, not to beat yourself up about past failures but to establish a starting point for moving forward. Then you can begin to make changes that will take you where you want to go.

Don't expect drastic change overnight, but recognize the value of any forward movement, no matter how small it seems at first. Many people fall into the trap of saying, "This is the year I'm going to eat healthy." "This year I'm going to lose weight." "This summer I'm going to exercise." "I'm going to stop working so hard." "I'm going to work on my marriage." "I'm going to enjoy my hobbies more."

All good things.

And all setups for failure.

Statements like these are pictures of where you want to be at some point in the future, but they are not goals that will change your behaviors. You get where you want to go one step at a time. Those steps, small though they may be, are what change your behaviors for the long term. Changed behaviors will take you where you want to go.

Behavior changes when you name the new habit.

What are you going to do? And how?

For example, suppose you have high blood pressure and your doctor prescribed medication, but half the time you forget to take it. You might say your goal is to "take my medicine." But you already know you should be taking your medicine, and you don't. Rather than state the obvious, ask how you can create a habit to take your medication consistently.

Suppose you decide, "I will take my blood pressure pill with my breakfast every morning." How are you going to make that happen? For instance, you might move your pill bottle to the kitchen and keep it next to the cereal bowls you use every morning, instead of stuck away in a bathroom medicine cabinet. You might use a weekly pillbox with daily compartments so you will know at a glance whether you have taken each day's dose. These are specific behaviors. Simple actions make a big difference, but first you must state what the simple action is.

Many parents discover this principle when they try to get young children to do something. A general instruction such as "Go clean your room" seems specific to the adult, but not to the young child. Twenty minutes later the exasperated parent discovers the child did nothing—or made the mess worse. What if the parent says, "First pick up all your toys and put them in the toy box, then put all your books back on the shelf"? Now the child knows what to do. The task is simple and specific.

Name the specific habit you want to form, and picture yourself doing it, one step at a time.

Behavior changes when you see progress.

If you had to drive from Chicago to Denver, would it be enough for you to just get in the car and head west? For some people, yes. They would enjoy the adventure, and they might arrive in Denver eventually. (Or they might unintentionally end up in Wyoming, or never see the end of Iowa.) More likely, you would look at a map. You would note the major cities along the interstate highway between Chicago and Denver, and you would judge your progress by approaching these cities, navigating through each one, and finally being on the other side. With each passing city, you would know you were that much closer to Denver.

Behavior changes need the same sort of landmarks. We're far more likely to make lasting behavior changes if we can mark off progress. It's difficult to go from a steady fast-food diet to "Eat healthy" in one fell swoop. If you're aware that you eat fast food an average of five times a week, perhaps your goal is to eat fast food no more than two times per week. Later you might change your goal to once a week, and eventually your favorite fast food becomes an occasional treat you don't have to feel guilty about.

Progress is something you can measure. Regardless of the goal you set, think about what you can count as you work toward your goal. Count the pounds you lose, or the laps you run, or the times per week you *don't* bring work home, or how many minutes you spend walking around the neighborhood after supper, or how many books you read in a month.

Rather than saying, "I want to read more," say, "I will read for half an hour before bed three times a week."

Rather than saying, "Get some exercise," say, "I will walk with the dog around the park and back every Monday, Wednesday, and Friday afternoon."

Behavior changes when you can see progress, when you can

look back at where you were and see how far you've come. Give yourself landmarks by which to measure your progress.

Behavior changes when you know what to do.

Verbs are the stuff of life. What are you going to *do*? How do you get from saying, "I'd like to go back to school so I can get a better job," to having that degree in your hand? How do you get from saying, "I'd like to be more involved in my community," to actually being involved in your community? How do you turn that new gym membership you paid good money for into an exercise plan?

Even the simplest aspiration will stymie you if you don't know what you're supposed to *do* to achieve it. A strong goal statement will have a verb at the core. It will map out what you will do and how often or by when you will do it.

"In the next thirty days, *identify* three schools that offer the degree I want."

"*Attend* next month's public meeting of the community action council."

"In the next two weeks, *experiment* with six different pieces of exercise equipment for thirty minutes each, and rank them in order of how much I enjoy them."

Break down big goals into specific action steps you can take within a definite period of time. Each action, when accomplished, leads to the next action statement that takes you closer to where you want to be.

Behavior changes when it's realistic to do what you plan.

"Do fifty chin-ups every workday morning."

"Read two books per week."

"Cook dinner every night from scratch instead of a box."

Are these goals specific? Measurable? Action oriented?

Yes. But are these doable? If you're starting from zero in these categories, then probably not. It's one thing to set a goal that challenges you, and it's another to set yourself up for failure. A strong goal will require a commitment, but it will be something you are capable of doing. If you're a chocoholic, "Stop eating chocolate" is probably not realistic, though you might set a goal that limits when and how much chocolate you eat. "No desserts" will not be as helpful as "Choose fresh fruit for dessert three times a week." A goal that stipulates "every morning" or "every day" most likely does not give you much grace for real life. The first morning you are not at the gym at 6:00 a.m. or the first bite of birthday cake at the office party makes you a failure. Why would you do that to yourself?

Set goals that challenge you and require change in your habits and behavior, but don't be so aggressive that you shoot yourself in the foot in the process. The point is to set goals you can sustain with more than a temporary burst of resolve. Do not compare your goals to someone else's. That just doesn't work. You don't have identical lives and temperaments. Goals for your own wellness have to be realistic in your life.

Behavior changes when the end is in sight.

Goals are not forever. If you're driving from Chicago to Denver, you will eventually get to Denver. From there you can decide if you want to continue on to Phoenix or Salt Lake City or some other destination calling your name at the time.

Set goals with a time limit, such as a few weeks or a few months. Make sure you allow enough time to actually change your habits, but then feel free to review and reevaluate. If a particular change in action gives you the results you want, you can decide to continue in that behavior for the next block of time, or perhaps even ask more of yourself. On the other hand, if the actions are not bringing desired results—if you are not more well than when you started—evaluate the goal, adjust behaviors, and give yourself a fresh start without recrimination.

Putting a time limit on goals does not mean you only have to endure that long and then you can revert to your old ways. The point is to allow enough time to actually change a habit, and to build in some specific times of evaluation so you can be sure you continue to move to a higher level of wellness. If you lose thirty pounds but your cholesterol or blood sugar levels don't come into healthy range, then perhaps you do need medication. Maybe you've been eating healthier food, but you're bored with the options and you'd like to find some new recipes before you're tempted to lapse back into old comfort foods. Perhaps in the course of accomplishing a goal, you discover something that is fun, and you would like to engage in that activity even more.

Set short-term goals for developing new habits, give yourself a small reward for accomplishing them, then set new goals and look forward to accomplishing those as well.

Set "SMART" goals.

The acronym SMART is popular among people who manage projects or work with goals in the business world. The origin is uncertain but goes back somewhere between thirty and fifty years. Over that period of time, business leaders and writers have adapted the acronym to a variety of settings and used the letters as a reminder of various words. The general usefulness comes as a quick, easy-to-remember checklist for goals that lead to getting things done or accomplishing change. What likely started in the corporate world has leaked into the lives of everyday people who just want to be sure they're staying on track with their goals. Words commonly used with the acronym include the following:

S = Specific, Simple, Significant
M = Measurable
A = Actionable, Achievable, Attainable
R = Realistic, Relevant
T = Timely, Time-bound

These words reflect the fundamental principles of changing behaviors and forming new healthy habits for wellness. Using SMART as a checklist, evaluate the sample goal statements below. Will these goals lead to changed habits? How would you improve on them?

- I will cut back on caffeine.
- I will cut back on soda to two cans per day for two weeks, then one can per day for two weeks.
- I will exercise an hour every morning before I go to work.
- I will walk twenty minutes three times a week on my lunch hour for six weeks.
- Make more time for my friends.
- Twice a week for the next two months I will invite a friend to coffee or lunch.
- I will eat more fruits and vegetables.
- For the next four weeks, I will write down the fruits and vegetables I eat each day to find out if I have at least five servings on an average day.
- I will talk to my doctor about my health.
- When I go to my physical next month, I will take a list of questions about my medications so I can understand them better.
- Enjoy myself more.
- At the end of each day for two weeks, I will write down three good things about the day.

- Find more balance between work and home life.
- For the next six weeks, I will begin each day with a to-do list to keep me from getting distracted at work.
- Spend more time with God.
- Write in a prayer journal three times a week for six weeks.

We're going to look together at each of the seven facets of the Model for Healthy Living that we use at Church Health Center Wellness: nutrition, friends and family, emotional life, work, movement, medical care, and faith life. At the close of each section, you'll have the opportunity to write a SMART goal to help you move along the wellness spectrum.

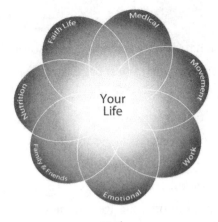

25

Nutrition: Food Is a Gift from God

Eating alone is dangerous to your health.

I ate at McDonald's for the first time in 1965 when the number of hamburgers sold was in the mere millions. I was ten years old, and the restaurant had recently opened in my neighborhood to great fanfare. I settled into a booth with my hamburger and french fries, and I gagged after two bites. They were terrible! The meat was tough and the french fries too salty. If only I had stopped for good then.

Like most Americans, if I am in a hurry, the Golden Arches or another fast-food restaurant lures me. It's convenient and satisfies my craving for fat and salt. I know what I am eating is not healthy. The density of calories, the concentration of cholesterol, sodium, and starch—it's not what my body needs. "You are what you eat" is true. There's no getting around it. And in America, with two fast-food restaurants on every corner, what we are is increasingly obese.

Since the proliferation of fast-food restaurants in the last twenty years, the number of obese teenagers has tripled. One in six teenagers is now obese. In the same time period, teenage consumption of soft drinks doubled. Fast-food restaurants sell high-calorie, sugary soft drinks often without even offering any healthier beverage options. The resulting explosion in childhood obesity made formerly unusual diagnoses of illness in children now commonplace. When I first began practicing medicine twenty-five years ago, it was rare to diagnose a child or teenager with hypertension or type 2 diabetes. Now it is not only common but almost a daily occurrence.

Is America's addiction to fast food to blame? It's hard not to see a correlation. Almost every child in America eats at McDonald's at least once a month. All the drive-through lines in the medical district where I work are backed up at lunchtime. Our national fast-food addiction has reached epidemic proportions.

Highly processed, refined foods are not only bad for our physical bodies but bad for our spiritual health as well. Fast food is perfect for eating alone and in a hurry—a formula for spiritual isolation. Eating alone is dangerous to your health.

Make mealtime relational.

For Jesus, the concept of fast food would be unacceptable. From the Gospels, we know that Jesus liked to have conversation with his meals. He used meals to create community. Eating was not something to do as quickly as possible; meals were intended to be time for fellowship, learning, and connection. Jesus ate at the homes of Pharisees and social outcasts. He made sure the masses who followed him had something to eat. He stayed with friends in Bethany and conversed with Mary while Martha fussed, probably about a meal. On the eve of his death, Jesus shared a meal with his closest followers, and John records for us at length the range of topics they talked about. After the resurrection, Cleopas and another unnamed follower recognized Jesus when they sat down to a meal with him. Later Jesus turned up on a beach and cooked breakfast for his disciples.

In the book of Acts, early Christians gathered to share their faith, eating a full meal together as a way of growing closer. Today we refer to this as slow food, but for early Christians, this was a part of their life and faith.

We can use mealtime to nurture community while nourishing our bodies. Following the path of Jesus and of those in the early church, we should cook and eat in community more often—families, friends, neighbors, church groups. Building connections over food, where we sit down and eat together, tends to make people less likely to rush off to the next thing. The benefit of the meal extends far beyond basic nutrition. Instead of eating alone at your desk, take your sandwich to the company cafeteria or to an outside picnic table and converse with others while you eat. Between afternoon activities and the evening rush, plan intentional time to eat together with your family, rather than picking up fast food or rummaging through restaurant leftovers in the refrigerator. Invite someone home for lunch after church on Sunday. Realistically, we'll all eat alone some of the time, but it doesn't have to be all of the time, or even most of the time. Shared meals may take more time, but they are spiritually enriching and healthier for our bodies.

Receive God's gift of food.

Food is a gift from God. Church Health Center Wellness has a vibrant children's program, Child Life Education and Movement. We teach children this fundamental attitude toward food even at the youngest ages. God created Adam and Eve and gave them a garden to live in—a garden rich with food. God said, "I give you every seed-bearing plant on the face of the whole earth and every tree that has fruit with seed in it. They will be yours for food" (Genesis 1:29). Right in the first chapter of the Bible, we see that food is a gift from God. Yet we treat it as a product of technology, and the physical need for it has become an inconvenience that gets in the way of our speed and efficiency.

Try asking a few kids if they know where their food comes from and see how many of them can get further back in the food chain than a box or frozen bag in the grocery store. Despite all the changes in food preparation and delivery that are supposed to make our lives easier, the fact remains that the most nutritious food we can eat is food closest to the source. Fresh, whole food looks much the same when harvested as it does when you bring it into your house. It hasn't been mashed or dehydrated or reconstituted or formed into something else. It doesn't have a long list of added ingredients on the label that requires a science degree to understand. It hasn't been through a series of machines intended to make it more appealing or convenient. It is what it is. Receive God's gift of food.

Children often need to taste a new food four or five times before they are willing to accept it into their palates and see it as an option they would select—or at least eat willingly—in the future. The earlier we introduce foods to children, the earlier they come to see them as choices. Adults are not patient enough with children or with themselves. Rather than offer a new food to children repeatedly and see what might happen over time, parents quickly resort to what they know kids will eat—even if it is processed, fried, and almost devoid of nutrients. And if adults taste something once and don't immediately like it, they see little reason to ever taste it again. At Church Health Center Wellness, we introduce new foods to children in fun ways, and often a child then introduces the food to the family.

Small changes make a big difference.

Everybody has favorite foods. Every family has the rice pudding, corn casserole, turnip greens, or pecan pie that shows up at holiday gatherings. Often multiple generations of family members have learned to prepare this recipe—with piles of sugar, butter, and salt.

If the food manufacturer didn't change the fresh, whole food into something else, we do it ourselves.

I'm not asking you to throw out your grandmother's favorite recipe. But consider whether you can make small changes to Grandma's turnip greens and have a tasty result without adding a pound of fat. Perhaps you can prepare a favorite recipe with half the sugar or salt and never notice the difference, but you won't know if you don't try. Perhaps you can bake or grill a favorite food and discover that you like it just as well as when you fried it, but you won't know if you don't try. At our Wellness center we run cooking classes where people learn about the simple changes they can make to favorite foods to prepare them in healthier ways without depriving themselves of the pleasure of eating them.

I am not a fan of fad diets. I'm not a fan of dramatic changes in eating patterns that people are not likely to sustain over time. I'm not a fan of punishing people with a limited diet. I'm not trying to help people eat differently for a day or two weeks or a month. I want people to eat for a lifetime. Certain foods give you a greater chance of being physically healthier over a longer period of time. We encourage people to eat in a way that gives them more energy now and more disease-prevention benefit in the long term. If people come from a culture featuring a certain kind of food that I personally wouldn't eat on a regular basis, we don't tell them they can't have it anymore. That won't last a week. But we will try to go over the recipe and suggest how to prepare it in a healthier way. Then we have a chance that change will be long-term.

Our attitude toward nutrition is "all things in moderation." Rather than promise yourself you're never going to eat your favorite foods again because you know they aren't healthy, put them in balance with an array of foods you know *are* healthy. Rather than adopt a diet that makes you feel deprived every minute of every day, focus on balance and moderation. Reduce your calorie intake by

300 calories a day and combine that with looking for reasons to take extra steps, such as parking at the far end of the parking lot when you shop. Small changes add up to better nutrition without turning your life inside out.

Nutrition is an important piece of wellness, but it is not the only piece. The point of better nutrition is to build healthy, strong bodies that lead to being whole people who are better connected to God. Food is God's gift to us, and caring for our bodies with nutrition is our gift back to God. Be grateful for God's gift and treat it with care.

Write a SMART goal for yourself in the area of nutrition (Simple, Measurable, Actionable, Realistic, Time-bound).

Explain how you think reaching this goal will contribute to your overall wellness.

_____

_____

_____

_____

_____

_____

_____

_____

_____

_____

_____

_____

_____

_____

_____

_____

_____

_____

_____

_____

_____

_____

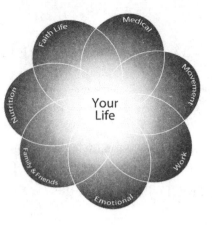

Your
Life

Faith Life

Medical

Movement

Nutrition

Family & Friends

Emotional

Work

26

Friends and Family:
You Don't Have to Do It Alone

Willpower is greatly overrated.

Michelle, twenty-one years old, tried to be sophisticated. She informed me her breasts were tender and she thought she had a bladder infection because she was going to the bathroom so often. Before I even walked into the exam room, though, the nurse made the diagnosis. A pregnancy test was positive. This was not good news for Michelle.

"I told him he could not get me pregnant! I didn't want to do it! I can't believe this happened!" And she began to cry.

I gave her a few minutes, then tried to be as positive as possible, beginning to talk about prenatal vitamins and an appointment with the obstetrician.

She interrupted me. "What if I don't want to have this baby? You must be thinking terrible thoughts about me and I can't believe I'm saying this, but I just can't have a baby."

I listened to her tell me everything that worried her, then said, "I want you to do two things before you make a decision. First, I want you to talk to your mother, and second, I want you to talk to our pastoral counselor."

Michelle was quiet.

"I can't tell my mother if I'm going to have an abortion," she finally said. "I can't even say the word." The wheels in her mind kept turning. "I know I'll hate myself, but it's what I have to do." And finally, "You're right. I'll talk to my mother."

It's okay to need help.

It's incredibly hard to live a healthy life all by yourself. I'm convinced that being healthy only occurs in the midst of a community. Having family, friends, coworkers, and fellow seekers of the life well lived is essential to optimum health.

Some will no doubt tell me, "All I need is willpower."

Willpower not to overeat. Willpower to exercise daily. Willpower to avoid excesses. Willpower to control spending. Willpower to— you fill in the blank.

In my opinion, willpower is greatly overrated. Few of us have the innate ability to do everything necessary for health on our own. We need help. We need others to encourage us when we despair, pick us up when we fall, and walk alongside us when we tire. We may succeed in the short term on our own, but in the long term we need a team.

New Year's is a popular time for athletic clubs to recruit new members. The entire population just gorged themselves into five extra pounds and examined holiday pictures that reveal what they actually look like. It's a perfect setup for making rash resolutions. Gyms often require people to pay a joining fee and guarantee a certain length of membership with monthly payments. The clubs make money because they know most people will not follow through with their resolutions to "get healthy," but the contract will require them to pay the monthly fee anyway. We return to our old ways mostly because our efforts depend on our own willpower. On the other hand, working toward better health as part of a community with others who have similar goals can improve your chances of success considerably. I've seen thousands of people change their lives because of the community they find at Church Health Center Wellness.

People depend on other people to experience the fullness and goodness of life. When God created Adam, God saw right away, "It is not good for the man to be alone" (Genesis 2:18), and God created Eve. From the very start, humans were in relationship with God and with each other. Christian monks used to go out into the desert alone in the third and fourth centuries. The theory was that without the distractions of the world—including relationships— they could devote themselves fully to God. Untold numbers of them returned after years in the desert and admitted the isolation did not bring them any closer to God. They missed the people they loved. Even Buddha had a similar experience. Total isolation did not lead to his goal of enlightenment. We need family and friends around us.

Can family and friends be trying? Yes. Can family members sometimes be destructive to wellness? Yes. Are there times you must pull back from a family member whose anger is so intense that it negatively affects your health? Yes. But in those situations you can find "chosen family." People with whom you don't share a family connection may function as brothers and sisters. With them, you share your intimate thoughts, laugh, experience the goodness of life. At the end of the day, you can just sit down and be yourself in their presence.

For good or for bad, children have their first picture of health and wellness in the family. If it's a dysfunctional picture, they'll have a lot of work to do later. But if it's a healthy picture, then they're on the road to wholeness.

At Church Health Center Wellness, we're educating children

to make healthy life choices even in the preschool years. With a foundational principle of respect, we teach them to be in community with one another. We're not a drop-off babysitting service. We have specific program times with specific purposes. Parents are required to be in the building while their children are in our program. They can plan their workout schedules around the programs they want their kids to experience, and we have a point of contact with parents both at drop-off and at pick-up. Whether a child attends a program on nutrition, physical activity, self-esteem, body image, safety education, or violence prevention, through the child we touch the family. We become partners with the parents in creating a picture of wholeness in relation to God for the children.

In Child Life Education, children begin making their own goals at age six. They learn early on that they have a voice in their own health and they are capable of making healthy choices. Our staff reminds children of their goals—"How are you doing with drinking more water?"—and reviews goals with the kids every quarter. We've been fascinated to see that children become agents of change in their families. They'll say, "I wish my mom wouldn't. . . ," or "I wish my dad would. . ." Because of how children feel about behaviors they know are not healthy, parents decide to change. Children see that their choices matter and that they can impact someone else's life as they live in community.

Nurture relationships before the crisis hits.

Nadine came to me with a number of significant health problems, but I was a bit confused about why she chose the Church Health Center. She worked as a dispatcher for the police department, which I knew was a fairly well-paid job and certainly offered health insurance. On our sliding scale, we would expect her to pay 100 percent of the cost of her visit. So I asked her why she came to us when her employer surely carried insurance.

Graciously, Nadine answered that she would understand if she could not be a patient at the Church Health Center, but she couldn't afford to pay for the insurance and private doctors.

I was still befuddled. As far as I could see, she lived alone and wasn't supporting anyone else. So with a good job, why couldn't she afford insurance?

Nadine explained that her daughter was a drug addict and years ago had a child diagnosed with an unusual disease at age three. Nadine cared for her seriously ill granddaughter until she died at the age of eleven. The girl never had health insurance, and her care generated an enormous bill—hundreds of thousands of dollars. Half of Nadine's income now went to pay the bills for her granddaughter who had died.

I offered to work with the hospital to ask them to write off some of the bills, but Nadine refused my suggestion. She explained that when she made that monthly payment, she did so with joy. Because of the doctors and the hospital services, she shared with her granddaughter eight cherished years she would not otherwise have experienced. Every time Nadine paid on the backbreaking bill, she remembered the immense joy her grandchild gave her. She didn't care how many years it would take to pay the bill, because she reveled in the gift of that child's life.

I assigned Nadine to the 10 percent bracket on our sliding scale. If a granddaughter with a serious, terminal illness touched her life so deeply, I could only imagine what Nadine gave to the girl's experience of love and joy during eight years of illness. We don't do it alone. We give and take in community with family and friends.

One of my best friends is a Jewish rabbi in Memphis. He has taught me an amazing amount about Jesus from a Jewish perspective. When I had joint replacement surgery, I saw Micah's security in the friendship he offers me. Day after day, I experienced the worst pain I ever remember. Micah came and sat on the side of the bed and for fifteen minutes sang Jewish prayers for healing. It was a powerful experience for me.

Where would I have been without my friend?

Where would the little girl have been without her grandmother?

These relationships began before crisis hit. In good times, it's incredibly important to nurture relationships that will sustain you in the dark night. You need people who will not give up on you when it seems like morning will never come. When doubt assails you, people who love you—and whom you love—can believe for you. Through them, you may see that the kingdom of God can prevail no matter what.

Jairus, a first-century synagogue ruler, asked Jesus to come and heal his daughter who was sick. Jesus was on his way when someone from Jairus's house arrived and said, "Your daughter is dead. Don't bother the teacher anymore." The people surrounding the girl gave up—for good reason, it would seem.

But Jesus had a kingdom perspective. He said to Jairus, "Don't be afraid; just believe, and she will be healed." And he continued walking toward Jairus's house. When he got there, he found a mob of people standing around pitying the family and crying over the situation. In spite of the mourners, and despite the report of the girl's death, Jesus carried a kingdom message of hope and support. He sent most of the crowd away. Perhaps they were mostly gawkers and not much real help. That happens in a crisis. Jesus, though, kept his focus on the girl's parents and his own closest friends. He gathered the inner circle—those who expected to see God's presence in the situation—and he brought the girl back to life (Luke 8:49–55).

God draws us into life and the goodness of life. But when we're in the midst of illness, pain, or suffering of any kind, it can be a mighty struggle to see the presence of God. One of the great points of comfort the New Testament offers is that Jesus himself struggled with suffering. He knew what was coming in his own death on the cross and prayed, "Father, if you are willing, take this cup from me" (Luke 22:42). An angel appeared to strengthen Jesus, yet still his anguish continued and he prayed "more earnestly."

When we look at the same events from God's point of view, we see God's ability to identify with us in our sufferings. Surely God's own suffering must have been intense when Jesus died. If a child dies, God's heart is the first to break.

A normal human response to suffering is to doubt, to ask questions, to wonder what's true. Doubt is a dimension of faith, not a failure of faith. Nobody needs to feel their faith is not as robust as someone else's because they have questions only God can answer and God seems silent.

Yet we should never discount the power of suffering to change our lives. Suffering has the power to effectively end the meaningful part of someone's life because the doubt is too dark, the questions too overwhelming, the answers too slow in coming. If you have not experienced this life-wrenching sort of suffering, you don't realize its destructive potential.

But.

But suffering does not have to win.

Anyone can come right to the brink of the abyss and wonder, *What if I just jumped?* But we stifle the impulse.

But we step back from the edge.

But we fall back into the arms of people who love us.

But we gather our wits and say, "What was I thinking?"

Not everyone gets to the "but," though. We don't get to the "but" by sheer individual willpower. I'm convinced that what pulls people back from the brink of the abyss is community. Knowing you don't have to face suffering alone is a game changer. When strength seeps out of your fingernails and you can't hang on any longer, you know the arms and hearts of others will catch you. Others will believe when you can't. Others will pray when you can't. Others will clench you until the terror passes and you savor God's presence again.

It's not too late to make friends.

Family and friends are crucial to your health, and you are crucial to theirs. You receive from the community you're part of, but you also contribute to it. Others offer qualities you need, and you offer qualities others need. Who are the people you depend on most, and what are you doing to strengthen those relationships? Who depends on you, and how are you responding to their needs?

Time together. Kind acts. Hilarious laughter. Shared joys. Encouraging words. Prayers and tears. True confessions. Silence together. Acceptance of the real you.

If you need help sticking to your exercise goals, family and friends can come alongside and encourage you.

If you need encouragement to cook differently, family and friends can share the experience with you.

If you're ill, if you're at your wit's end with your job, if your feelings are so scrambled that you can't make a simple decision, family and friends can help, through both presence and action.

If this piece of your overall health is missing, it's not too late to surround yourself with people who care for you, and to offer relational care to others. Do this now, apart from a crisis, and a community of family and friends will be a springboard of hope when you need it most.

Write a SMART goal for yourself in the area of friends and family. (Simple, Measurable, Actionable, Realistic, Time-bound).

_____

_____

_____

_____

_____

_____

_____

_____

_____

_____

_____

_____

_____

_____

_____

_____

_____

_____

_____

_____

_____

_____

_____

_____

Explain how you think reaching this goal will contribute to your overall wellness.

_____

_____

_____

_____

_____

_____

_____

_____

_____

_____

_____

_____

_____

_____

_____

_____

_____

_____

_____

_____

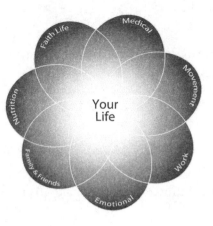

27

Emotional Life:
You're Supposed to Feel It

Stress is going to happen. It just is.

Maria, the young mother of a two-year-old, came to see me because she had discomfort around her pelvis. At first it seemed like a simple bladder infection, but the more questions I asked, the more I saw she did not have the typical symptoms. Instead, she talked about vague pains in her abdomen. Slowly the real problem emerged. Two months earlier, Maria had a miscarriage, and she had not been the same since. A physical exam was normal, as I suspected it would be. Her profound sense of the loss of her child manifested in a physical sensation, but she was not medically sick.

Ricardo's mother brought him in because he was a ten-year-old complaining of pain in his chest. At first I thought she was afraid he might have a heart problem, but she asked me, "Do you think he needs to cry?"

I was confused, to say the least.

His mother explained, "Last week an older boy stole his new bicycle from him at gunpoint."

Feeling sick for Ricardo, I turned to him and asked, "How old was the other boy?"

"He's thirteen," he replied. This told me it was someone Ricardo knew and it could happen again.

I didn't know what to do except reassure his mother that Ricardo would be okay, at least physically. Did I think he needed to cry? I suppose so, but I doubted it would make his problem go away.

Emotions are the real deal.

An incident from my third year of medical school has stayed with me for decades. Another student was presenting a patient, and she began telling about the patient's family and social situation. The attending physician interrupted and said, "You've crossed the boundary and let yourself get too close to this patient."

Doctors are trained to keep emotional distance from patients. The truth is, no one needs to learn how to be distant. What we need to embrace and teach is how to get close to another human being. Patients are connected, body-and-spirit, so why should physicians pretend they aren't? I can't imagine treating patients such as Maria and Ricardo and not feeling their suffering. And on the flip side, I couldn't keep being a doctor if I didn't have a group of patients who feed me emotionally. They care about me and I know it. I hope they know I care about them.

I feel sorry for the person who controls emotions so tightly that he or she does not feel moved by the laughter of a small child or the stunning palette of a sunset, or who can't shed a tear when someone dies. Squelching your emotions is not a sign of strength. In fact, I think it's a weakness. Emotions are part and parcel of our body-and-spirit humanity. We need to better understand their place in overall health.

Emotions are complex responses to specific triggers. A certain scent takes you back to your grandmother's living room, and the memory may pleasantly calm you or agitate you, depending on your childhood experience of your grandmother's living room. You hear an edge in someone's voice and instantly feel defensive because your father used that tone when he was angry. Your child smiles and your heart utterly melts. A teacher says, "Take out a piece of paper," and your stomach knots up because you're not ready for this pop quiz. Lunch with a friend who truly understands you keeps you flying high for days.

Life is full of emotions, some of them joyful, some of them stressful. Whatever they are, we feel them in our bodies. Heart rates quicken or slow. Muscles tense or relax. Eyes widen or close. Shoulders rise or slump. Feet dance with energy or drag with despair. Emotions of joy, success, satisfaction, love—these feed us. But life is also full of experiences that drain us—feelings of failure, broken relationships, unfair accusations, insane workloads, children who go astray. A frightened ten-year-old's chest hurts, or a grieving mother feels her empty womb. Simply being poor can be devastating to the spirit, yet our health care system does not recognize that emotional and spiritual suffering can lead to physical illness.

For good or for bad, emotions affect our moods, and moods affect our judgment. This includes the decisions we make about wellness and health. Emotions can mean the difference between mixing up a crisp, colorful salad or reaching for the bag of cookies. Emotions can mean the difference between going out with friends you enjoy or couch-slouching for six hours. Emotions can mean the difference between enjoying your work or dreading the next encounter with your boss. We all have our ways of coping with painful emotions. Some push discomfort on to someone else with an aggressive comment and pay the price in that relationship. Some avoid talking about what disturbs them and hope that makes it less real, though it doesn't. Some partition off pain and continue on with the motions of the rest of their lives, never acknowledging how unresolved emotions affect everything they do. Some set out to determine by trial and error exactly how much chocolate it would take to make them feel better!

Stress is going to happen. It just is. Coping by making healthy choices instead of indulging old habits begins in understanding what triggers your feelings and owning up to the ways you have coped in the past.

Take out the trash.

You don't have to fight every battle. You don't have to be "right" in every encounter that pushes an emotional button in you. Sometimes you can walk away and be better off for that choice. The battles worth fighting are the ones that bring you joy and love and drive you closer to God. Ultimately, these are the only things that matter. Bridges burn quickly. Before you take on an endeavor that potentially could harm an important relationship in your life, ask yourself, "Is it worth it to use up what I have in the bank with this person on this issue?" When you stop to think, it's amazing how many things won't matter in two hours or two weeks. Save your emotional energy for things that do matter because they deepen your experience of joy and love.

Take out the trash on a regular basis. What happens if you don't take out the kitchen trash when the bag is full? It overflows. It stinks. It makes a mess that didn't have to happen. The messier it gets, the less you want to go near it. Cleaning it up becomes more work than simply taking the bag out in the first place. The same is true of emotional trash. Instead of getting rid of it on a regular basis, we let it overflow until we can't stomp another item into the can. The whole mess explodes in our faces, and now we're scraping stuff off the walls.

How do you take out the emotional trash? Exercise is a big first step. Exercise improves mood and calms physical reactions to stress. And then talk to someone trustworthy. Depending on what your trash is, you may or may not have a friend who can help you take it out. You might need to talk to a pastor, a counselor, or another confidential professional who can hear you speak the truth about your life without your worrying that this person will repeat what you say to anyone, judge you, or hand you pat answers. And then keep your eye on the trash can and don't let it get so full. Empty the trash on a regular basis before it gets stinky and explosive.

Life is possible.

Jill, twenty-one years old, was about to start a new full-time job that also would give her the health insurance she needed. To celebrate on the morning of her first day, she went for a horseback ride with a couple of friends. Something spooked her horse; it started bucking and Jill fell off. However, her booted foot snagged in a stirrup, and the horse dragged her for fifty yards before finally stepping on her shoulder. Jill was conscious and screaming the whole time, and some onlookers responded rapidly. One was a trained emergency medical technician who recognized immediately that Jill needed an airlift, not an ambulance.

During the night, doctors told Jill's parents they would have to amputate her leg. Because of a rare condition, the leg had been a problem for Jill's whole life, so at first she thought perhaps it was just as well to be done with it. Before long, though, she realized this was not going to be easy. Phantom pain was persistent. She couldn't work. Visits from friends dropped off. Getting out of the house seemed like more trouble than it was worth. So she stopped going out, stopped even trying to reclaim the life she had looked forward to before the accident.

Because Jill technically had not started the new job, the insurance had not kicked in. This left her floundering for the medical care she needed. Further expensive surgery was inevitable to relieve painful pressure on her sciatic nerve, requiring both an orthopedic and a vascular surgeon. An orthopedist offered to help her for free, but the vascular surgeon would not take her on. Prosthetics are costly, but without one Jill had no option but crutches. Eventually she received a prosthetic on loan, but it had been made for a much older woman, did not fit well, and was only a temporary solution. By this time she was on seven different medications. All this stress took its toll on Jill's emotions, and she became clinically depressed.

Then someone told Jill about the Church Health Center and she came to see me. I was glad to be able to help her medically by arranging her surgery and coordinating her care, but I also pointed her to our Wellness facility. She went through the door of Wellness with her mother just to find out what I was talking about. On that first day, an exercise class was beginning and she was invited to join. She went back. And she went back again. The community and encouragement Jill found at Wellness began to turn her around emotionally. She made friends, exercised, talked, and began to see that life was possible after all. One by one she went off her medications except for one to manage her phantom pain. We arranged for a custom-made prosthetic for Jill, and four years after the accident, she renewed her hope of having a job and independence.

"The Wellness center is what made me see that life would go on," Jill says. She now gets out of the house regularly, is far more social, and has returned to sunbathing and fishing, activities she loved before the accident.

Emotions are important to a full, rich life. Jill certainly experienced the whole spectrum. By God's grace, she discovered that the draining emotions that so easily arise from suffering did not have to control her life. It was possible to find joy and love and be close to God. Today Jill has a tattoo on her shoulder, right in the spot where the horse stepped on her and left a permanent horseshoe-shaped impression. It says, "For when I am weak, then I am strong" (2 Corinthians 12:10).

Write a SMART goal for yourself in the area of emotional life.
(Simple, Measurable, Actionable, Realistic, Time-bound).

_____

_____

_____

_____

_____

_____

_____

_____

_____

_____

_____

_____

_____

_____

_____

_____

_____

_____

_____

_____

Explain how you think reaching this goal will contribute to your overall wellness.

_____

_____

_____

_____

_____

_____

_____

_____

_____

_____

_____

_____

_____

_____

_____

_____

_____

_____

_____

_____

_____

_____

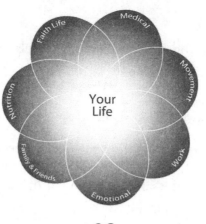

28

Work: It's One Piece of Meaning, Not the Whole Ball of Wax

It's not the quantity of life that matters; it's the quality.

Milton was a hardworking man. The calluses on his hands were so thick they felt like sandpaper. He was seventy-nine but still worked every day on his small farm.

"I get short of breath," he told me. "It's never been this way before."

"When was the last time you saw a doctor?" I asked.

"I went once when I was fifteen."

He denied having chest pain, but his shortness of breath convinced me to do a treadmill test to look for coronary artery disease, which could lead to a heart attack.

To my astonishment, his treadmill test was completely normal. "Did you get short of breath while walking on the machine?" I probed.

"Why, shoot, that was nothing."

I was perplexed. His symptoms still concerned me, so I gave him nitroglycerine tablets. The next time he had symptoms, I explained, he could put one under his tongue. He readily agreed to try this, and I waited for him to come back.

"Well, did the nitroglycerine help?" I asked.

"Naw," he drawled, "didn't make a bit of difference. I still get out of breath just like before."

I was confused, but thankfully this time his niece was with him.

"Uncle Milton," she said, "did you tell the doctor you only get short of breath when you haul concrete up the hill to build onto the back of your barn?"

"No," he said, "but what difference does that make? I've always been able to do it before."

He was completely serious, but my concern for his heart vanished in an instant. Instead, I wondered whether a man half Milton's age could do what he was doing at seventy-nine.

"I think your heart is fine," I said.

"But what about my breath?" he demanded. "What am I supposed to do?"

"Maybe you can get someone to help you with the concrete work."

"Do you know how much it costs to get good help these days?"

There was no reasoning with him.

Mr. Lucero was a Filipino immigrant who arrived in the United States at age seventy-four speaking almost no English. He had worked his whole life, and there was no way he was going to come to a new country and sit around and do nothing. So he got a job cleaning tables at McDonald's. One day he was walking to work and got hit by a truck. By all rights he should have died, but ambitious doctors used every trick of technology at their disposal and snatched him back from the hands of death. For more than three months he was on a ventilator, and he would have to live the rest of his life with a tracheostomy, a hole in his neck to get air to his windpipe. But miraculously, he survived and eventually left the hospital. He can't stand up, mentally he's not the same, and he has to put a finger over the hole in his throat to talk. When he came to see me after all this, his first words were, "When can I go back to work?"

Menachem is a young African American man who grew up in Tupelo, Mississippi. He was born at the time of the Camp David Accords, and his mother was so enamored of the prospect of peace in the Middle East that she was determined to name her son Anwar, Jimmy, or Menachem. The family was poor, but Menachem turned out to be a gifted football player and earned a scholarship to Rhodes College in Memphis. He played hard and studied hard, with the dream of going to medical school. He didn't get in the first time he applied, so he became a clinic assistant at the Church Health Center. That's how I met him. He worked forty hours a week for us, and he had a second job as a bouncer at a nightclub. One Sunday night my wife and I ran into him in a record store, which turned out to be his third job. Mary and I fell in love with Menachem and took him under our wing.

When Menachem got into med school, I sat down with him and said, "You realize you can't work while you're in med school." I'd been to med school. I knew the realities.

He answered, "But I've been working since I was eleven."

"What did you do when you were eleven?"

"I collected garbage on the back of a truck before school."

Menachem's work ethic never ceases to amaze me.

Work is a gift.

We are made to work. Even before God made Eve, and before the fateful decision to eat fruit that was off-limits, God put Adam to work. Genesis tells us, "The LORD God took the man and put him in the Garden of Eden to work it and take care of it" (2:15). Work is not punishment. It's a gift from God starting at the time of creation. God intended for humans to be productive, and the value of work is intrinsic. If you let people determine the value of your work based on how much money you earn, you're missing the point. God does not put monetary value on your work. Plenty of people make a lot of money, even enormous amounts, but their work doesn't draw them closer to God. In fact, it may pull them away from God.

On one end of the spectrum are people for whom work is a means to an end. Get a paycheck and spend the money to make yourself happy, whether that means the simple security of paying your bills or the luxury of buying the latest gadget or taking a dream vacation. But if that is all your work means to you, then you're wasting one-third of your life, and your eyes will be closed to the presence of God in your circumstances.

At the other end of the spectrum are people who become slaves to their work. They take it with them everywhere. They think about it all the time. They marginalize family and friends. They trivialize nutrition and exercise, all for the sake of working more. If work becomes your god, it separates you from God who created you and loves you.

There must be a happy medium. It's not the quantity of life that matters; it's the quality. It's not the quantity of income that matters, but the quality that healthy attitudes toward work add to your life.

You don't have to be a doctor or be doing something incredibly creative in order to enjoy your work. I see patients who make minimum wage and love what they're doing. They love talking to people they encounter in the course of their work. They love feeling productive and seeing the tangible result of their work. They love providing a service someone else needs. Keeping another person's house, hauling garbage, mining coal, providing childcare—these are not glamorous jobs. The people who do them may not even receive what I would consider a fair wage, but they're not bitter because they understand the dignity and value of work in itself, not because of what society says it's worth in annual income.

God is present in your work.

You may be in a dream career and love your work.

You may feel trapped in a job you hate because you need the paycheck—or the insurance.

You may be just starting your working life and considering your options, or you may be reflecting on several decades and evaluating your choices.

You may feel isolated at home with children or an elderly parent who needs care.

You may be making more money than God but feel fundamentally unhappy.

You may be making next to nothing but sleep in sound satisfaction every night.

I'm not going to tell you there's a right or wrong answer about finding a job where you belong at this season in your life. I don't think there's a magic formula. But I will emphasize that work is only one piece of the meaning of your life. It's not the whole ball of wax. It's not even the main thing. Because money is attached to our work—and we need money for basic needs—we lose sight of the fact that work has no greater value in overall health and happiness than any of the other elements of healthy living. Whatever your work is, it's not separate from spirituality. It's not only for the sake of your body. Your work intersects with nutrition and movement, with family and friends, with your emotional life, and with medical needs. God is present in your work circumstances, and your work is an integral part of your experience of God.

I once presided at the funeral of a controversial, polarizing Memphis politician. All his former political adversaries came to the funeral. People from the left, people from the right, people who supported him, people who opposed him—they were all there. Many of them were now in their eighties. I listened to them talk and heard them say things like, "What was it we used to disagree about so much?" They literally could not remember what the animosity was all about. They knew they didn't like each other, but they weren't sure why. Finally, like old warriors, they came together and put the past behind them and enjoyed the present moment.

Don't wait until you're eighty for that perspective. Don't spend decades working and then look back and wonder why you thought it was so important to chase a particular position. Don't allow your work to consume you to the degree that you miss the river of beauty flowing through your life. Don't look back and regret that you were not fully present in the work you had at various seasons in your life because you pined for something else. Don't regard work as punishment or something to escape and miss the ways it can enrich your life and your connection to God.

Work is a gift from God. Receive it with gratitude.

Write a SMART goal for yourself in the area of work
(Simple, Measurable, Actionable, Realistic, Time-bound).

_____

_____

_____

_____

_____

_____

_____

_____

_____

_____

_____

_____

_____

_____

_____

_____

_____

_____

_____

_____

Explain how you think reaching this goal will contribute to your overall wellness.

_____

_____

_____

_____

_____

_____

_____

_____

_____

_____

_____

_____

_____

_____

_____

_____

_____

_____

_____

_____

_____

_____

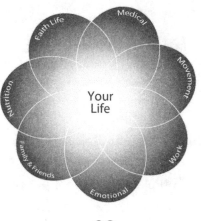

29

Movement: It's God's Design

Sedentary is not how God made you.

We are created to move. We have bodies with arms and legs and elbows and knees and fingers and toes. Our body parts bend, stretch, rotate, twist, swing, swivel, sway, pivot, and roll. We have joints and muscles and ligaments and tendons. Blood pressure and equilibrium constantly adjust and readjust to the needs and demands of movement. Our bodies are designed to move efficiently. And since we can't separate our bodies from our spirits, we, as whole beings created and loved by God, are made for movement. Watch an athletic competition or any form of dancing, and you'll see the beauty of movement and what our bodies can do—and the emotions and connections we express through bodily movement.

In the earliest pages of the Bible, we read about God walking in the Garden of Eden in the cool of the day (Genesis 3:8). God took an evening stroll! Even small children instinctively understand God's gift of movement. Babies thrash their legs and wave their arms, and their brains build synapses that bring purpose and control to their movements. They roll over, sit up, pull up, and walk. Children learn to skip and run and pedal bicycles and turn cartwheels and somersaults.

God created us to move.

We make it hard to exercise.

Nevertheless, we've built a society and infrastructures that get in the way of movement. Workplaces and shopping centers and churches and medical centers are miles away from where we live—sometimes many miles—so we rely on cars to get from place to place. Suburban houses feature oversized garages—often attached at the *front* of the house, of all places—as a reminder that our lives revolve around convenient transportation. Densely populated apartment and condo buildings go up in places with heavy traffic and no sidewalks. It's too far to walk to do an errand, and too unpleasant to walk for the sake of walking in the areas where many people live.

And we've gotten quite accomplished at excuses for not exercising.

"I can't get off work."

"I'm too tired when I get home."

"I just had my hair done."

"Between my job and my kids, I don't have time."

"Exercise is boring."

"It's too hard."

"My neighborhood is not safe."

"I can't afford a gym membership."

"I'm too old."

"I'm too fat."

"I don't have a weight problem."

"It makes me hurt."

"I start, but I can't stay motivated."

All this adds up to a split between people who do exercise and people who don't. Those who exercise have their own subculture of workout language and machines and shoes. Entering a gym can be intimidating to the uninitiated. "Movement" becomes exclusive rather than inclusive. It's an industry that requires money to participate, rather than a natural response to the way we're made. In response, more and more people are content to say, "This is how God made me, so I don't have to exercise"—even if they are morbidly obese or have a chronic medical condition that exercise would help manage.

This is not how God made you. No one who is physically active in any significant way will be morbidly obese. Simple low-level physical activity helps to manage a range of conditions. Rejecting physical activity is not part of God's plan. Sitting behind a desk all day and never getting up is not God's design. Parking yourself in a recliner to watch four hours of television before you drag yourself to bed is not God's design. Sedentary is not how God made you. God made you to move.

We don't value exercise as critical to our body-and-spirit existence. Over and over, we communicate that the brain matters more than the body. People whose livelihood depends on being smart in a cerebral way generally earn more money than those whose work involves physical labor. School districts under financial pressure eliminate physical education, sending the message that it was somehow an add-on in the first place, rather than a valuable part of the education process for the whole child. Memphis city schools, for instance, cut physical education because of finances, even though children who live in urban settings rarely have the option to simply go outside and play or join a soccer league. If you're not any good, you can't get on an outdoor basketball court. Kids go home, sit on the couch, and eat chips. We need creative ways to get kids active and moving, and we need to understand that physical activity levels *do* affect classroom learning.

Exercise is about more than weight.

The health benefits of movement—even small amounts—make up a long list. Exercise is not an optional category for healthy living. Exercise is not just for the "in" crowd who can afford to do it with style. Levels of physical activity affect all areas of our lives. The first benefit that jumps to mind, of course, is weight management. We all know we have to eat less and move more to combat weight gain. The average adult gains three or four pounds every year, and obviously this adds up over the decades. Typical weight gain for women going through menopause is fifteen pounds. We do have to be mindful of the relationship between exercise and weight. But beyond burning calories, physical activity carries many other benefits as well.

Exercise improves mood. Physical activity gets the brain chemicals churning, and you'll feel happier and more relaxed than if you don't exercise. You might yell at your kids less. You might be less annoyed with the self-centered coworker. You might tend more toward kindness, patience, and gentleness because you went for a brisk walk and you're in a better mood. Physical activity is probably the best thing you can do for yourself if you're feeling depressed, especially if you struggle with ongoing depression. When you feel anxious or depressed or stressed, working out may be the last thing you feel like doing, but it would be the greatest gift you can give yourself.

Exercise promotes sleep. If you have a hard time falling asleep on a frequent basis, or find that you wake up during the night and can't get back to sleep, you probably don't need a sleeping pill. You need more physical movement during your day. And better sleep improves your concentration during waking hours, makes you more productive, and keeps you in a better mood.

Exercise boosts energy. That might seem like a contradiction in terms, but it's true. Physical activity delivers oxygen and nutrients to your whole body. When your heart and lungs are doing their job well, you'll have more energy for the things you like to do.

Exercise combats disease. High blood pressure. Diabetes. High cholesterol. Osteoporosis. Arthritis. Regular physical exercise is a key weapon in preventing common conditions that lead to serious illness, such as cardiovascular disease. It also helps manage chronic conditions so they don't control your life.

Exercise makes you feel better about yourself. Meeting even small goals for exercise can boost your confidence. Getting in shape can make you feel better about yourself in general. Exercise distracts you from a vicious cycle of worries and negative thoughts. Exercise gives you the power to do something positive to manage your life.

Doris was an extremely likable woman in her midforties, with dark, shining skin, a pleasant smile, and warm eyes. But she seemed alone and defeated to me. She was easy to talk to, but it took awhile to figure out why she came to see me. It came down to, "I'm tired." She was on the verge of her seventh attempt to break her crack addiction.

"There is nothing you can tell me that I haven't heard before," she said to me. "I know I have to do it myself. I'll do anything to have my life back, but I've said that before. I've lost my job, I've lost my family, I've lost everything that was any good about my life."

I rolled my stool over to her and held her hand. After a minute, I said, "Why don't you come to our exercise classes? You can exercise instead of smoking crack."

She smiled. "That's a new one. It's worth a try."

She was desperate to feel better about herself, and I was pretty sure exercise would help and the class members would provide an accepting group to belong to.

Move more than you do now.

Deconditioning did not happen overnight, and physical conditioning will not return overnight. If you're just starting out on the exercise journey, the goal is not to turn you into an Olympic athlete or a leading contender in the local bodybuilding competition. The first goal is simply to move more than you do now—and enjoy it.

If you usually just let the dog out into the backyard, grab a leash and walk Fido instead.

If you usually look for the parking spot closest to the mall entrance, choose one at the far end of the parking lot.

If you usually push the button for the elevator and stand there and wait, take the stairs.

If you usually drive your car through the car wash, get out the hose and wash it yourself.

Walk to the mailbox to drop your bills in the slot.

Dig up your backyard and make something beautiful out there.

Take your kids to the park and push them on the swings and merry-go-round. Race them from one post to the other.

Put up a hoop in the driveway and challenge your child to a game of HORSE.

Get off the bus one stop early and walk the rest of the way.

Stand up and move during television commercials—but not toward the fridge!

Get up from your desk every two hours and take a lap or two around the perimeter of the floor where you work. Look out the windows and remember the world is there.

Clean your windows.

Clean your carpets.

When you finish lunch, walk for ten minutes before you go back to your desk.

Walk while you pray, and don't stop until you've prayed for everyone on your list.

Opportunities for increased movement are everywhere. Open your eyes and see where they are in your life. Exercise doesn't have to be something you hate, and it doesn't have to demand another continuous hour in your day that you simply don't have. Ten minutes three times a day brings plenty of benefits. Most important, you don't have to dislike the activity for it to count as exercise. If you're moving, it counts. The key is to find something you enjoy enough to make it a habit.

Do you enjoy movement more if you're outside? Do you enjoy exercise that's also a social opportunity, such as team sports or a walking partner? Do you like to crank up the music and move to the beat? Do you like the gratification of something that results from your effort, such as a garden of summer blooms? Are you more likely to be consistent about exercise at a certain point in your day?

Incorporating movement into our lives is not a one-size-fits-all proposition. I have forms of movement I enjoy, and you have forms of movement you enjoy. Certain situations deter me from exercise, and others deter you. The challenge is to know yourself well enough to identify what keeps you from moving, and what kind of activity would remove the barrier.

Then set reasonable goals. When you accomplish a small goal, set a more ambitious goal. You don't have to start with walking five miles a day, though eventually you might surprise yourself and be able to do it.

A mother brought her daughter to our Wellness center. The little girl was blind and in a wheelchair because of a deforming disease. "Do you think there's anything you have for her?" the girl's mother asked. "She gets bored throughout the day."

Kimberly, who runs our children's program at Wellness, took the girl around and explained the various options.

"I want to dance," the girl said.

Kimberly was unfazed and began to work with this child who wanted to feel her body move. Several months later, I walked by the dance studio and there she was, all by herself, dancing in her own way.

Remember that small changes bring big results, so even small efforts add up. Remember that exercise is not only about your weight, but also about wellness in all the dimensions of your life. Remember that God designed you to move.

Write a SMART goal for yourself in the area of movement (Simple, Measurable, Actionable, Realistic, Time-bound).

_____

_____

_____

_____

_____

_____

_____

_____

_____

_____

_____

_____

_____

_____

_____

_____

_____

_____

_____

_____

_____

Explain how you think reaching this goal will contribute to your overall wellness.

_____

_____

_____

_____

_____

_____

_____

_____

_____

_____

_____

_____

_____

_____

_____

_____

_____

_____

_____

_____

_____

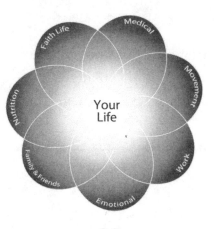

Your Life

30

Medical Care: Rewrite the Contract

God is smarter than any doctor.

I just don't think you're listening to what I'm telling you." Claudia was ready to fire me as her doctor, even though we met only moments before.

She started to cry. I stifled a sigh. We both were frustrated. She struck me as demanding, and I suspect she thought I was uncaring about her many physical symptoms. I tried to regroup.

"Let's start over," I said. "Tell me what makes you feel so bad."

Claudia looked up, and for the first time, we connected. Over the next several years, we came to understand each other, and despite our rough start, she seemed to believe I was the only doctor who actually did listen to her. Claudia had a serious liver disease and required a transplant. Because of the gravity of her disease, I enlisted several specialists to help with her care. Whenever one of them suggested a new drug, she asked me if I thought she should take it. On several occasions I had to leave the room and go look it up because I had never heard of it. I repeatedly said, "Claudia, I'm a family practice doctor. I don't treat a problem like yours every day. You have to trust the specialist's opinion."

And she would reply, "But you know me and listen to what I say."

Together we walked a long way from where we almost parted company.

Launch a partnership with your doctor.

Like it or not, we're all going to die. We live in a mortal coil and our days are numbered. Our bodies break down, and we must embrace that life includes medical needs. In the context of healthy living, medical care is only one piece of the puzzle. Good medical care doesn't make you healthy in isolation from other elements of healthy living. You're the expert on you and in charge of your health. The doctor—and the health care system—is your partner, not your driver. The doctor's role is not to tell you what's wrong with you, but to be a coach in helping you live a healthy life. The doctor sometimes will take on the role of a technician in helping you understand a particular condition or procedure, but decisions about health should always be yours. You don't ever have to say, "Whatever you think, Doctor," without having a clue what the options entail. Because of education and training, your doctor is your advocate and advisor, but the doctor is not God. God is smarter than any doctor. We are body-and-spirit beings created and loved by God, and health care starts there. If your doctor does not approach your medical care as a partnership in the context of your whole life, then fire your doctor. Plenty of good ones out there are waiting for you.

When people talk about doctors as a class of people, they make hostile comments. Collectively, doctors are a suspicious bunch. But for the most part, when people talk about their own doctors individually, they claim to like them. When you need a specialist, ask your primary care physician. Don't try to pick a heart specialist from the yellow pages. A good family doctor is going to point you toward other doctors who see the world the same way he or she does, including the specialists you need. The tricky part is finding a family doctor who wants to be your partner. I realize finding a doctor can be a minefield, but try asking your friends. Find out who among your family and friends has an ongoing positive experience with a primary care doctor. That's a good place to start for taking control of the medical piece of your own overall health care.

If you need a medical procedure, don't hesitate to ask questions. "How many times have you done this procedure?" is a reasonable first question. Sometimes you need a practitioner with experience more than you need a comforting bedside manner. If you're having surgery, you want the guy who has done it a thousand times, even if you don't like his personality. Don't hesitate to ask, "What is the complication rate? What is *your* complication rate?" Surgeons and hospitals keep those statistics. If a doctor is not prepared to discuss them, you probably want to talk to another doctor. Nobody should ever be reluctant to ask for a second opinion, and if a doctor is reluctant to send you for one, part ways.

Give and expect respect.

At some level, most doctors would like to feel they are partners with their patients. Healthy partnership requires mutual respect, but several prevalent attitudes can get in the way of respect in a medical setting.

The doctor's office is not the fix-it shop where patients can drop in when something breaks and expect the expert to fix everything—or come in with a list of twenty maladies to cover in a routine fifteen-minute office visit. Some conditions are the result of life choices you make, and only you can change them. If you're not willing to do some work, the doctor can't do much to help. At the other end of the spectrum, certain conditions inevitably lead to serious disease and even death. While doctors will offer the best medical care possible, they cannot alter physical reality no matter how insistently a patient demands they "do something." In a respectful partnership, the parties understand the strengths and limits each brings to the medical challenge. Expectations should be reasonable for the circumstances.

The doctor also is not an ATM for prescriptions. If you plan to come back next year when the pharmacy once again informs you they cannot refill the prescription, but in between, you do whatever you want as long as you have the pills, then you're not treating your doctor as a partner. In a respectful partnership, the parties take responsibility for their actions. If you're expecting the best from your doctor, make sure you're giving the best as well.

The doctor is not your Internet backup. You can find anything on the Internet. Just because it's on the Internet doesn't make it true, and it certainly doesn't mean it's true for you. Doctors see patients every day who read something on the Internet and now they're convinced they have a dreaded disease that explains mysterious symptoms they didn't even realize they had last week. I'm not kidding. It's also common for patients to read about a particular medication and become convinced it is causing an uncomfortable or dangerous side effect even before seeing the doctor—who may have another explanation to suggest. The doctor spends valuable time explaining why you don't have an obscure disease, instead of talking with you about what might really be happening in your body or in your life. In a respectful partnership, the parties seek the best of what each can give. Your doctor has training and experience, and you know the ins and outs of your own life. Bring the two together in the best way possible. The Internet probably is not it.

And the doctor is not a coffee klatch. Sometimes the best way to show respect *for* your doctor, and to create an atmosphere of respect *from* your doctor, is to get to the point. Your doctor doesn't need a long explanation of how you went to visit Aunt Jenny's farm for her forty-second anniversary so she wouldn't be lonely since her husband died two years ago—it was so sudden, who knew?—and while you were there, you decided to walk the dog, and the dog saw the postman, and you remembered Aunt Jenny always said the dog never liked that postman, and the dog started chasing the postman and pulled you into a ditch, and you turned your ankle. Tell your doctor what happened, but perhaps don't start that far back. Answer questions directly with clear information

A healthy partnership recognizes what each party brings to the table. You are responsible for your own health. Your doctor can't control everything you do. Your doctor is willing to help you if you're willing to help yourself. If you're worried, I'm worried. But if you don't care, how can I? Most doctors would be more inclined to put their time and effort into people who want to get better, rather than those who don't.

Other than in an emergency, the patient controls far more than the doctor. For instance, one of the biggest reasons medications don't bring desired results is that patients don't take them properly—or at all. You're a grown-up. I can't *make* you take your medicine. I can't make you play basketball instead of video games, or eat an apple instead of an apple pie, or work things out with your brother instead of letting unforgiveness fester. A partnership with your doctor means you hold up your end of the bargain and come to the health care table ready to make choices and take action. Remember, many people can be your companions in the process of following through on those choices.

Seek abundant life.

A woman in her early forties came to see me and casually mentioned she had noticed a lump in her breast. I did an exam and found she had a mass of at least ten centimeters in her right breast. I had no doubt it was cancer and told her so, then talked about treatment options. She said she wanted to think about it. A couple of days later, she returned and announced she had claimed her healing. She was certain God would heal her and she did not need to do anything medically.

"I do believe God will be with you," I said, "but the way to healing is surgery."

She wouldn't have anything to do with it. She wanted to do literally nothing about the growing mass. Over the next year, she came to see me on a regular basis. The tumor kept growing and finally erupted through her skin, but still she refused any medical treatment. She was 100 percent convinced God had healed her. We had one theological discussion after another, but she never would let me do anything for her other than change dressings and help contain the unrelenting oozing.

Eventually the tumor grew into the main artery in her chest wall and one night she bled to death. I have never fully known what to think about that.

On the one hand, I grasp fully believing that God will heal. My patient was incredibly at peace with her decision and never faltered, though she was an extreme case in claiming healing for cancer. More often I hear patients tell me they have claimed their healing over high blood pressure, diabetes, or other diseases that take a toll over time and can lead to stroke or heart attack. In order to prevent that progression, however, you have to participate in your own care—diet, exercise, medicine, therapies, treatments. Often people will see those actions as a lack of faith. Their logic is that if they truly believe God will heal, then they should do nothing at all. To do anything would mean they don't genuinely have faith God will heal. On the other hand, the New Testament encourages us to use the best medical techniques available. We are expected to use our brains and the tools God provides.

I also hear patients say, "It's God's will. This is the hand God dealt me and I will do the best I can with it, but who am I to fight God's will?" I counter with the conviction that God's will is for you to live a full, abundant life in God's kingdom. Surrendering to disease that can be managed with simple actions, or not taking advantage of available medical treatments for something more serious, means walking away from the full, abundant life. I don't believe that's faithful living that brings you joy and love and drives you closer to God. Medical treatments will not solve every problem, and I'm not talking about the extreme cases where it truly is time to let go. I'm talking here about conditions for which doctors can offer help in partnership with the choices patients make. Healing comes from God, but doctors and patients working together have a greater chance of revealing God's movement in the circumstances than passively doing nothing.

Be an active partner.

Medical treatment is not the answer to everything that goes wrong in your life or in your body, but when you hold it in balance with all the other elements of the Model for Healthy Living—nutrition, family and friends, emotions, work, movement, and faith—it plays an important role. The key is for you to actively participate in your medical care as a partner with your doctor. Claudia made me stop and listen, and we went on to have a fruitful doctor-patient partnership for years. If you don't feel you have a partnership with your primary care physician, you can take steps to change the situation. Hold up your end of the partnership and your doctor will more than likely do the same.

Write a SMART goal for yourself in the area of medical care (Simple, Measurable, Actionable, Realistic, Time-bound).

_____

_____

_____

_____

_____

_____

_____

_____

_____

_____

_____

_____

_____

_____

_____

_____

_____

_____

_____

_____

_____

_____

_____

Explain how you think reaching this goal will contribute to your overall wellness.

_____

_____

_____

_____

_____

_____

_____

_____

_____

_____

_____

_____

_____

_____

_____

_____

_____

_____

_____

_____

_____

_____

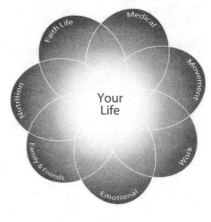

31

Faith Life: Don't Wait for a Crisis

The last time I checked, you cannot MRI somebody's spirit.

Marsha's arm was broken, but not badly. "How did it happen?" I asked.

"I pushed a child out of the way of an oncoming car, but the car hit me instead."

I acknowledged the brave act. "That was a kind thing you did."

Marsha didn't see it that way. "I was watching out for a kid, but God should have been watching out for me. So where was God?"

That's a question I discuss often in my Sunday school class and one I suspect many patients have, but none had ever put it to me so bluntly. I didn't have a quick and satisfying answer. I was fairly sure Marsha would not have been comforted by, "God was watching out for you and your arm got broken anyway," which is what I believed. Instead, out of my own uneasiness, I shifted to a safer topic: casts.

Faith matters.

In the last hundred years, Western medicine has moved so far away from seeing faith as part of health that most of the time faith does not even arise in a discussion of healthy living. But it's critical. Half the patients doctors see come in because their lives are falling apart—they have no specific physical problem. The last I checked, you cannot MRI someone's spirit. If we are not nurturing our spirits and working to create a healthy spiritual life, we will not be healthy physically and certainly not be healthy, whole persons.

At the Church Health Center, we see people from all over the world. One of my patients was an eighty-two-year-old immigrant from Thailand. Speaking almost no English, she came from a tiny rural village to an overwhelming urban setting. Fairly soon after joining her children in the United States, she developed a significant heart problem. We were able to take care of it, but then she had a brain tumor. While we were sorting out whether it made sense for her to undergo surgery for this tumor, I admitted her to the hospital for tests. In the middle of the night, a nurse telephoned.

"You have to come and do something about your patient. She's sitting in the middle of the hall in the lotus position, chanting."

I can understand this caused some consternation in a hospital setting, especially since no one was on hand to communicate with her through her own language. So I called the woman's grandson to see if he could help get her back in bed. But I also understood my patient was expressing her Hindu faith and believed faith and wellness were connected. That much she got right.

In the Christian tradition we turn to prayer at such moments. Prayer is perhaps the most obvious and outward expression of faith that God can move even in difficult circumstances. But what do we expect when we pray for healing?

A doctor would consider a patient healed when physical symptoms improve and laboratory tests show a return to normal ranges. This may not always be what we mean when we pray, though. For a child hit by a car and now in a coma, we might pray for the child to be completely restored to normal function and live a long and healthy life. If we are praying for an eighty-year-old man in a coma, however, we don't expect him to return to youthful vigor, but we might want him to walk again. Or do we simply ask that he not suffer? Do we ask that he die peacefully and his family be comforted during the loss? Healing services have found life in churches across the denominational spectrum, and understanding what healing means also is on a spectrum. Regardless of what we hope and pray for in various circumstances, I believe we can expect five things when we pray for healing.

Healing will always be a mystery. No one can ever say what constitutes healing or when it occurs. Healing and its definition seem to be one of those things only God truly understands. And it's okay if we can never explain it in rational terms.

Illness and suffering can be a way to grow closer to God. In the midst of experiencing pain, it might be hard to see how suffering allows us to identify more closely with the wounds of Christ. The plain fact is sometimes suffering blinds me to the presence of God in the moment. Then again, it may be the very thing that gets me to see that the suffering servant whom Isaiah preached about—Jesus—is the very way God brings redemption to the world.

Life and death are in God's hands. Science and medicine are pathetically limited in what they can achieve. In almost every situation, the complex and restorative power of God's creation of the human body determines whether we are healed. The remedies medicine offers are at best a gentle aid in the process.

God cares about our suffering. Prayers for healing should always remind us that we are not alone. When the woman touched the hem of Jesus' robe, he felt her pain and sought her out. When his friend Lazarus died, Jesus sobbed.

God will not abandon us. When the psalmist walked through the valley of the shadow of death, God was present. In prayer, we expect to experience God's redeeming presence, even if physical healing does not come.

Hardly a day goes by when a patient does not ask me to pray. Sometimes I'm not sure what the patient is really asking of me, but I believe the power of prayer for healing is real and is the underpinning of all we do as we seek to be healing communities of faith.

Prayer shawls are tangible, heartfelt symbols of the prayers we offer in faith for healing. A simple Internet search on the term will turn up more links than you can click. People in churches all over the place are knitting and crocheting prayer shawls. Most of these people have no idea of the Jewish background of a prayer shawl. They're just knitting shawls for people who are sick and want these people to know someone is praying for them. Churches in Memphis supply prayer shawls to the Church Health Center, and on a nearly daily basis a group of staff prays over a shawl designated for a specific person. The staff would never think of giving out the shawl without this time of prayer.

The healing benefits of the prayers may be mysterious, but I do think the physicality of the shawl, and knowing someone knitted it and others prayed over it, brings comfort. I have seen this in stoic men who you'd think never in a million years would sit under a shawl. But when I go to see them, there they are, with the shawl on their laps or around their shoulders.

Find your own expression of faith.

At Church Health Center Wellness, we encourage our members to cultivate a life of faith. We don't say, "This is what you have to do," or "You have to believe this way." We don't advocate a particular theological perspective. We simply believe that if you ignore your faith life, even if everything else is perfectly in sync, you will be out of balance. God's love is so great and broad and bold that it can encompass an array of ways to be faithful to God's call. Faith you practice in times of wellness and balance will yield well-formed habits to lean on in times of illness and crisis. So don't wait for the crisis to find your connection to God.

During my second year of seminary, I fell under the spell of Henri Nouwen, a theologian and writer on the subject of the spiritual life. I talked with him a few times about what I wanted to do with my life and asked for his help in fully discerning my future. He suggested I should go to France over the Christmas break, to the Taize community. During World War II, Brother Roger hid Jews from the Germans, and after the war he created an interdenominational community built around reconciliation. It turned into an ecumenical monastery with members from Catholic, Orthodox, and Protestant traditions. Taize developed its own distinctive style of worship focused on prayers and a unique musical style. I knew little else about Taize, but if Henri Nouwen said I should go, that was enough for me. I made arrangements for the first week of January and flew to France.

I went for a week of silence in a house with twelve other people. Three times a day we ate a bowl of soup. Twice a day we went to chapel services. Once a day, we spoke individually with one of the brothers who belonged to the order. The rest of the time, we were in silence. For many people, this would be a highlight of the spiritual life. This creative, amazing community is the setting for powerful religious experiences.

Not for me.

It was January and the house had no heat. I was freezing cold every minute of every day. I was hungry the whole time. My bed had only one thin blanket, and they made you wake up at a ridiculous hour. The winter days were short and the nights long. I just did not connect with the brother to whom I was assigned to talk once a day. My room was under the stairs, about seven feet by eight feet in size, with a bed on the floor, a small desk, and a chair. They discouraged visitors from reading books while they were there, instead pointing to the meditative experience.

For seven days I was thoroughly miserable.

It was something to remember once I got home, but I have no interest in returning to a week of cold, hungry silence. As romantic as it might sound, it's not for me. I might even wish I was the sort of person who could make that work, but I know I'm not. The great lesson from the experience, though, was that there is not one right way to connect to God. I had to find my own way of hearing God speak to me, and you have to find yours. If it doesn't come from being in silence, that's okay. If it comes through noisy, active involvement in a cause or mission, that's okay. It can come through any kind of music, any form of prayer, any style of worship, virtually any activity. What's important is that you seek to be connected to God.

Being connected to God is not an intellectual undertaking, meaning that you get all the right theological pieces in place and then you're all set. It's a life undertaking, a habit, a discipline that comes through regular, faithful practice. A healthy faith life often gives people the courage to eat right, move more, restore relationships, find meaning in work. Faith drives us to the ultimate goal of being in communion with God, and from that perspective we see the whole, full, abundant life God wants for us.

Write a SMART goal for yourself in the area of faith (Simple, Measurable, Actionable, Realistic, Time-bound).

_____

_____

_____

_____

_____

_____

_____

_____

_____

_____

_____

_____

_____

_____

_____

_____

_____

_____

_____

_____

_____

_____

Explain how you think reaching this goal will contribute to your overall wellness.

_____

_____

_____

_____

_____

_____

_____

_____

_____

_____

_____

_____

_____

_____

_____

_____

_____

_____

_____

_____

_____

_____

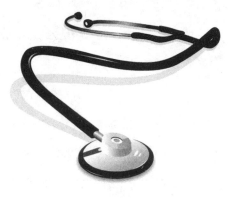

32

Share Your Vision of Wellness

*Being broken doesn't prevent us from helping
each other move toward health.*

Sharon runs support groups at Church Health Center Wellness. In a group for weight loss, she asked participants to write down their wellness visions. "Where do you want to be as far as wellness?" she asked. "How would you look? How would you feel? What would you be able to do? Where would you be? What actions could you take to move in that direction? What support do you need?" As Sharon took the group through the questions one at a time, she stressed that this wellness vision was a personal document. No one else was going to read it, including her.

To Sharon's surprise, the group members were eager to share their visions. They clambered to turn in what they wrote to Sharon or read aloud to each other. In particular, James wanted to tell the group what he wrote down. James had a creative bent and was an artist and knitter. He came to Wellness nearly every day. James explained he lived his wellness vision every time he came through the doors. He shared greetings with people he liked, he attended cooking classes, he exercised. James said he got "cheer bumps" all over his body just thinking about the community he experienced at Wellness.

In our wellness coaching model, health coaches meet with members once a week for six months. They talk about a wellness vision and three-month goals at every visit. For some members, it's difficult to verbalize what they want for themselves because they haven't always had the option to pursue such personal goals. Their lives are crammed with caring for others, putting out fires, and lurching from crisis to crisis, and their own goals take a backseat. In health coaching sessions, individual members have a companion on the journey, someone who knows the road well and is sure of the destination.

At Wellness, support groups abound, from weight loss to diabetes management to breast cancer survivors. Members can pause long enough to put into words what they're working on, what they're hoping for, the picture of wellness they want for themselves. In community they remember they are not alone, and in community they remind each other they are body-and-spirit beings created and loved by God.

Learn to spot wholeness around you.

"Me and Thee" is not the answer to anything. I don't claim to know the mind of God, but I do know that the greatest insights into what God wants for me come from a community of people who are also searching for some of the same things I long for. When I tap into the resources they offer me, I have a greater chance of heading down the right path. Writer and theologian Henri Nouwen gave us the concept of the "wounded healer." We are all broken in one way or another, but that does not prevent us from helping each other move toward a better sense of wholeness and health. We may all be broken, but our brokenness does not keep us from being part of the healing process for someone else. We all can help each other see the vision of wellness God wants for us.

Whoever you are, when you are part of a community, you have something to contribute as well as something to gain. Over the years, I have been the doctor for many elderly African Americans who grew up picking cotton in northern Mississippi or western Tennessee. These are all people who, at various points in their lives, endured the worst America has to offer. They grew up in the Deep South during the extremes of racial segregation. Strangers, or people they barely knew, treated them with disdain. Yet they worked hard and went to church every Sunday. Most of them are the age of Martin Luther King Jr., and some participated in the civil rights movement. One or two actually were garbage workers during the garbage workers' strike that led to King's assassination in Memphis in 1968.

What fascinates me about almost every person with this background is a remarkable lack of bitterness. In fact, rather than observing bitterness, I witness just the opposite. They share a common refrain I've come to expect when I greet a patient who is elderly and African American. I ask, "How are you?" and the inevitable response is, "I am fine and blessed."

Fine and blessed. How do you get to be fine and blessed when you have nothing? When life has been unfair and unkind to you? Fine and blessed when in a capitalistic country you have no capital? Not only do you have no money, but you have very little social capital. It is not unusual for these patients to have families that take advantage of them. Their children have stolen from them or abused drugs and expected their parents to bail them out of jail. Still, without any hint of irony, they continue to see themselves as fine and blessed.

I have come to regard this mind-set as a form of spiritual capital. In fact, when I see certain people on my patient list for the day,

I make sure I give myself time to discuss not only their physical problems, but also their views on life. I spend ten minutes listening to their hearts with my stethoscope and ten minutes listening to their hearts with my soul. I want to learn from them how one comes to be "fine and blessed." What do they know about life that I do not know? I can assure you that most of my friends or the people in my church do not see their lives as fine and blessed.

All my patients who see themselves as fine and blessed came to this way of living on their own without any planning. They had no intentional desire to embrace life in a manner different than people who experience life in a less fulfilling way. Too many people are unhappy, unfulfilled, lonely, and without joy. They are a long way from being fine and blessed. But what a marvelous perspective the "fine and blessed" group offers for the rest of us. Imagine having people with this outlook in your life on a regular basis. My patients who say "fine and blessed" to me are sharing their picture of wholeness, and it's one I can learn from no matter what is going on in my life.

Share your picture of wellness.

Whether or not you create a written document, I encourage you to put your picture of wellness into words. This may be a phrase or a sentence with which you encourage yourself. It may be brief answers to the questions Sharon asked the weight management group. The same questions apply to any facet of wellness that may be most challenging for you right now. Remember to identify your strengths as a starting point, rather than making a beeline to problem areas. The Model for Healthy Living includes seven elements: nutrition, family and friends, emotional life, work, movement, medical care, and faith life. In which of these areas do you have strengths? How can you use these strengths to move you toward your overall picture of wellness? Life is about what is working, not what is broken. You can't build on a pile of rubble. You have to find solid ground.

Then share your vision of wellness. If you're in a support group, share it there. If you have a few close friends or trusted family members, share it with them. If you're in a group at your church, share it there. Invite people to walk beside you on the road ahead. The journey will be all the richer for having someone with you, and the benefits of taking the journey together will multiply for you and those who travel with you.

Finally, live your vision of wellness. Surround yourself with the virtues of Colossians 3: compassion, kindness, humility, gentleness, patience, forgiveness, and the love that binds them all together. Treat others with the virtues. Treat yourself with the virtues. As you make goals, move toward them, reach them—or sometimes lapse— let your life reflect these characteristics of God.

The kingdom of God is God's picture of wellness—complete health, wholeness, connection to God. It's God's reality, and God invites you to be part of it. Jesus brought this reality of wholeness to our broken world and our broken lives. Health care you can live with—wholeness of body-and-spirit—will take you toward the wholeness God offers to you.

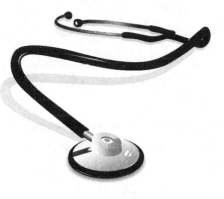

33

Do It for the Ones You Love

"Blessed are the poor in spirit,
for theirs is the kingdom of heaven."

The first time I met Ora, she was pleasant and friendly. She was easy to talk to and answered all my questions directly. Her problems were straightforward—hypertension and diabetes—so the office visit was quite ordinary. As I prepared to leave the room, things took a turn and a moment later Ora left a lifelong imprint on me.

She asked, "Do you mind if I bless you?"

I looked at her, eyebrows raised.

"I like to know my doctor has the Lord looking out for him," she explained.

No patient had ever offered to say a blessing over me before, but how could I refuse? And why would I?

"I would be honored," I answered.

Ora shot out of her chair, grabbed my head with both her hands, and pulled me to her bosom. With the voice of a revivalist, she called out, "May the Lord anoint you with the Holy Ghost and may all the healing power of the Lord Jesus Christ descend upon you and remain with you from this day forward." Then she pressed her hands firmly against my head, lifted my chin, and directly peered into my face. "I am so happy to have a Spirit-filled doctor. I knew it the moment I laid eyes on you."

I swallowed and stammered, "Thank you. I will see you back in three months." Doctors like to think they are in charge during office visits, but clearly I was not.

After that, whenever Ora came, I was ready for my blessing. She always considered herself one of God's chosen. Her father sharecropped for a living and Ora was one of ten children. Chopping cotton was her assigned work, though she liked picking better. "We didn't have much," she said, "but we had Jesus."

Ora made it through the tenth grade and then her oldest son was born. She married a few years later, had more children, and moved to Memphis, where she worked as a housekeeper for a wealthy family in town for fifty years. During these years, she raised her own children and several generations of the family she worked for. Her oldest son came home from the war in Korea and was never the same mentally. He began drinking and abusing drugs and eventually paid the price with his life. Ora was heartbroken, of course, but she never rejected her son for his decisions. "You can't judge someone until you walk in his shoes," she told me. "No matter what he did, he was still my son."

Her daughter's story is remarkably different. Ora worked two jobs to make sure her kids finished high school. Shirley, the baby of the family, received a four-year scholarship to the University of Tennessee at Martin, then attended law school, became a public defender, and eventually won an elected position as a criminal court judge. Shirley and her husband are in a position to take Ora on a trip each year, and one year they traveled to Israel. Ora could hardly contain her enthusiasm as she told me about this adventure. She splashed in the Sea of Galilee and strolled the streets of Nazareth, but her unparalleled joy was singing in Jerusalem.

"They took me to this cathedral where everyone would sing out with praise to Jesus, so I sang, 'Holy, Holy, Holy, Lord God Almighty.' It was beautiful for me to be there."

Then Ora reached into her purse and pulled out a vial. "I can't leave today without anointing you with this olive oil mixed with water from the Jordan River."

It was time for my blessing, and I was pleased to receive it. Ora opened the bottle and poured the oil in her hands, then made the sign of the cross on my forehead and on the backs of both my hands. "I am blessing your hands," she explained, "because throughout the day you will be touching other people like me, and I want you to pass this on." Then she placed both her hands on my head and said a prayer.

Now she does this every time she comes. I'm ready for my blessing from Ora. I need my blessing from Ora. Then I go and find a staff member who I think needs a blessing. I grab someone and push the person into the exam room and say, "This is Ora. She's here to give you a blessing." Certainly the circumstances of Ora's life through the decades brought more than her share of privation and adversity, but she intentionally steers toward the joy and takes others with her.

"Blessed are the poor in spirit," Jesus said, "for theirs is the kingdom of heaven. Blessed are those who mourn. . . . Blessed are the meek. . . . Blessed are those who hunger and thirst for righteousness. . . . Blessed are the merciful. . . . Blessed are the pure in heart. . . . Blessed are the peacemakers. . . . Blessed are those who are persecuted because of righteousness, for theirs is the kingdom of heaven" (Matthew 5:3–10).

These famous verses from the New Testament, which we call the Beatitudes, begin and end with the kingdom of God. Jesus' coming to our world announced that the kingdom of God was here. He burst through brokenness and turned everything upside down and inside out. The kingdom reality that Jesus lived and preached—and in which he healed—grabbed people and pushed them toward the blessing they needed. It still does today. Body-and-spirit wellness is possible in the here-and-now kingdom of God.

The people who influence and support you on your journey to wellness may come from unexpected places, as Ora and so many other patients have done for me. Be open to how God will move in your life as you seek to move closer to God in your pursuit of wellness. Wholeness is not so much about being disease free as it is about experiencing the sacred in your life every day. Health care is not about technology, pills, or money. It's about people. It's about you. It's about the people in your life. Whatever becomes of the health care system as an industry in the United States, you can take charge of your own health.

Steer toward the joy and take others with you. Do it for the ones you love.

Coming Soon

From Dr. Scott Morris's
Church Health Center Team

40 Days to Better Living

A series of practical books
dealing with specific health issues

You want to feel better—and *40 Days to Better Living* provides clear, manageable steps to get you there, through life-changing attitudes and actions. If you're ready to really live better, select one or more elements of the 7-step Model for Health Living—Faith Life, Medical, Movement, Work, Emotional, Family & Friends, and Nutrition— and follow the 40-day plan to improve your life, just a bit, day by day. With plenty of practical advice, biblical encouragement, and stories of real people who've taken the same journey, this may be the most important book you read this year!

Bimonthly release schedule, beginning July 2011.

Titles to include:

Optimal Health / Hypertension / Depression / Smoking Cessation / Weight Management / Stress Management / Aging / Addiction / Diabetes / Anxiety / Caregiving

Available wherever Christian books are sold.